The Paleo Cookbook for Two

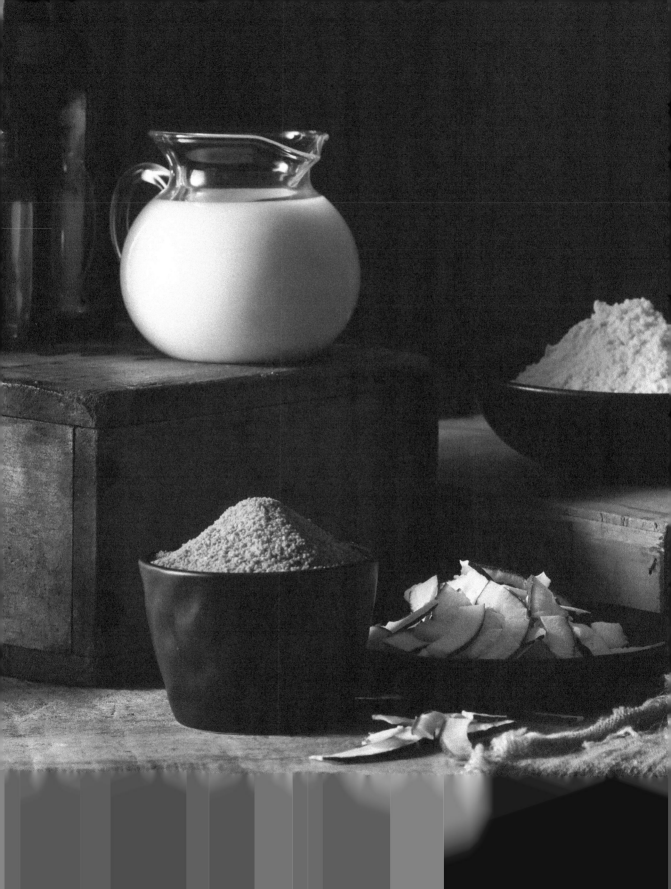

The Paleo Cookbook for Two

100 Perfectly Portioned Recipes

Ashley Ramirez, PhD & Matthew Streeter

Photography by Elysa Weitala

ROCKRIDGE PRESS

For general information on our other prod-ucts and services or to obtain technical support, please contact our Customer Care Department within the United States at (866) 744-2665, or outside the United States at (510) 253-0500.

Rockridge Press publishes its books in a variety of electronic and print formats. Some content that appears in print may not be avail-able in electronic books, and vice versa.

TRADEMARKS: Rockridge Press and the Rockridge Press logo are trademarks or reg-istered trademarks of Callisto Media Inc. and/or its affiliates, in the United States and other countries, and may not be used without written permission. All other trademarks are the property of their respective owners. Rockridge Press is not associated with any product or vendor mentioned in this book.

Interior and Cover Designer: Gabe Nansen
Art Producer: Sue Bischofberger
Editor: Claire Yee
Production Editor: Andrew Yackira

Photography © 2020 Elysa Weitala, with food styling by Victoria Woollard.
Ashley Ramirez's author photo courtesy of Olivia Reed Photography; Matthew Streeter's author photo courtesy of Andrew Hall Photography.

ISBN: Print 978-1-64739-735-7
        eBook 978-1-64739-437-0

R0

To Raleigh, Mama loves you.
To Lu, Daddy loves you.

Contents

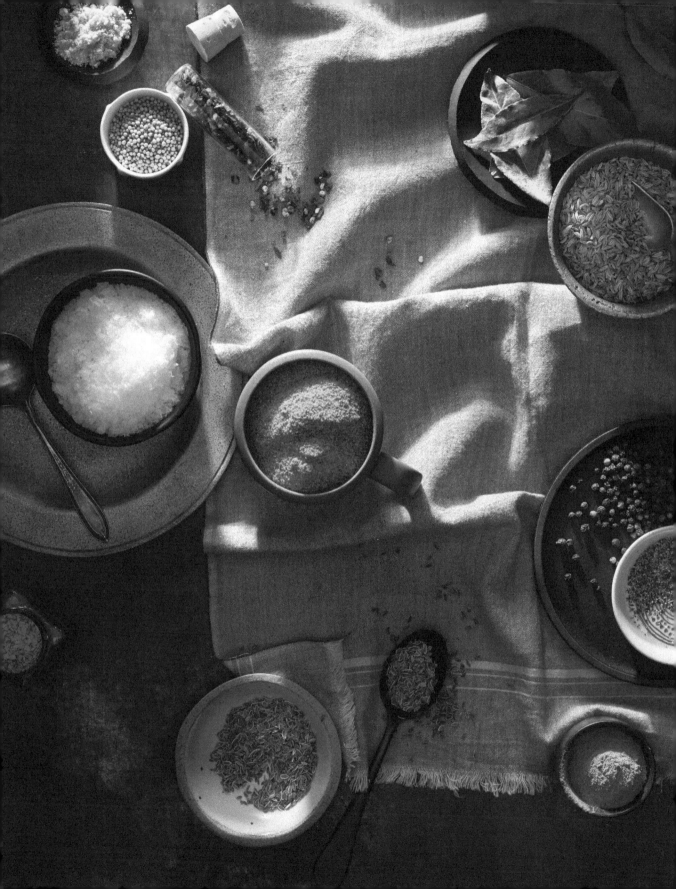

Introduction

Hello! Matt and Ashley here. Thank you for buying our book. We cannot wait to share with you 100 Paleo recipes designed for two people to cook and share together. Some of these recipes have been enjoyed by our customers at Mason Dixon Bakery and Bistro for years and some are brand new, created just for this book. Here, we will teach you what Paleo is and why we feel it is the best nutrition lifestyle for your health and overall well-being. Along the way, we also include tips to help you be successful with the Paleo lifestyle and point out common pitfalls that can cause people to falter.

There are a variety of recipes in this book, geared toward both new and seasoned home chefs. While we are well versed in the culinary field, we didn't start out that way—we all begin somewhere, and we can always learn more. We use this approach at our restaurant and are always looking for ways to improve recipes and incorporate different ingredients. We have also included a wide selection of vegetarian dishes, because it is completely possible to follow the Paleo diet without eating meat. Look for the labels under each recipe title to quickly find the vegetarian options.

Cooking for two can come in many forms, but it should be fun. Whether with your partner, child, roommate, or friend, there are ways beyond eating to work together in the kitchen. Cooking requires planning, shopping, prep, cooking, and cleanup, in addition to eating. We'd like to challenge you to rotate roles and responsibilities with your cooking partner and allow yourself to leave your comfort zone. The recipes in this book are designed to serve two people, but many can be scaled up for leftovers or to serve a larger group. Be it two people, or ten, these recipes are certain to excite your taste buds and nourish your body, leaving your heart and mind satisfied.

So what are you waiting for? Let's dive in and get cooking.

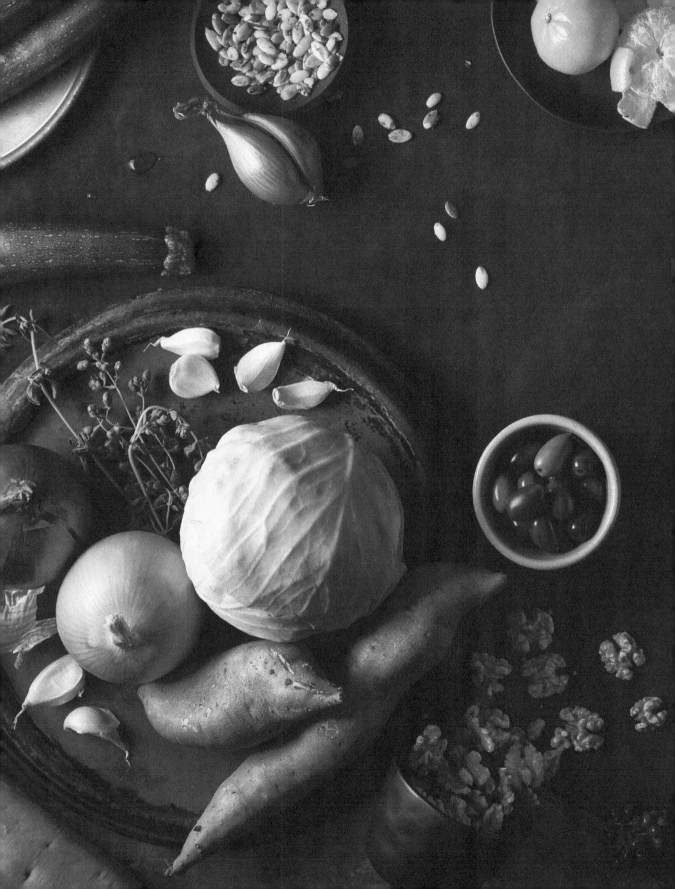

CHAPTER ONE

How to Eat Paleo

—◇—

When switching to a Paleo lifestyle, it's important to understand what you should and shouldn't eat. In this chapter, we'll discuss the modern American diet and how it differs drastically from Paleo, and we'll offer a guide for how to structure your plate for maximum health benefits.

If you're first starting out with Paleo, you likely have some questions. For instance, many newcomers wonder why Paleo omits grains if we've historically been told to make grains a central part of our diet. They also wonder how to replace grains. Others wonder how they can enjoy different cuisines and keep their meals interesting while also using Paleo-friendly ingredients. These questions and more will be answered in this chapter to set you up for success on your Paleo journey.

What Does "Paleo" Mean Exactly?

The Paleo diet is often referred to as the "caveman diet" or "stone-age diet," but what does this really mean? During the Paleolithic era, one's diet consisted of items that could either be *hunted* or *gathered*. Lean meats and seafood were *hunted*, while fruits, nuts, seeds and vegetables were *gathered*. Following a "Paleo" (short for Paleolithic) diet refers to returning to this basis of food consumption, eliminating highly processed and commercialized nutrition found on grocery shelves today. The idea is to focus on foods that our bodies are naturally able to utilize as fuel.

When determining whether an ingredient is Paleo-friendly, the first step is to ask yourself, "Is it made by nature or by machine?" The next step is to determine whether the ingredient is only available because of modern farming practices. Modern farming practices introduced ingredients like wheat, corn, dairy, and legumes, and they also allow for genetic modification.

When we think of food as fuel, it's easy to see why a nutrition plan based on high-quality, all-natural ingredients caught consumers' attention quickly. Early on, the Paleo diet was heavily popularized among athletes, but it soon spread to a wider audience due to its reported health benefits.

Paleo's Health Benefits

Focusing on only Paleolithic and natural foods allows us to eliminate highly processed foods from our diet, producing an array of health benefits. Commercially, the most attractive benefit of the Paleo diet is weight loss. On the Paleo diet, weight loss is caused by an optimized distribution of protein, fat, and carbohydrates. Eating carbohydrates increases insulin in our bodies, causing us to crave more carbohydrates: The more carbs you eat, the more carbs you crave. Higher insulin levels cause our body to depend on carbohydrates as an energy source instead of fat. This leads to the storage of fat cells, resulting in weight gain. This becomes a vicious cycle that can be difficult to break. The Paleo diet helps by eliminating processed sugars and many high-glycemic foods, disrupting the cycle of reliance on carbohydrates. Once we break the cycle, the body can burn through stored fat cells for fuel, leading to weight loss.

One less apparent—but equally important—health benefit of the Paleo diet is the elimination of inflammatory foods. We often think of inflammation as an acute stress response to promote healing: A simple example is when we get a cut and blood rushes to the wound so a scab can form. But inflammation can become chronic, causing your body to live in a constant state of stress. Chronic inflammation can cause your body to attack healthy cells, potentially leading to an array of autoimmune diseases, including heart disease, diabetes, cancer, and more. Certain foods such as sugar, trans fats, and simple carbohydrates (those lacking in fiber) are known to increase the inflammatory response. The Paleo diet eliminates foods that can cause inflammation and focuses on foods loaded with vitamins, minerals, and antioxidants.

SAD: An Appropriate Acronym for What We Eat

———————— × ————————

The Standard American Diet (SAD) really is quite sad when we compare it to diets in other parts of the world. The SAD, also called the Western pattern diet, is characterized by high consumption of red meat, dairy, processed foods, and artificially sweetened foods with minimal consumption of fresh fruits, vegetables, nuts, seeds, and lean proteins. A 2016 study published in *Biomedical Journal* found that nearly 60 percent of America's caloric intake on average comes from ultra-processed foods, such as chips, crackers, soda, desserts, and candy. It follows logically that the United States has one of the highest adult obesity rates in the world. While diet is not the only contributing factor here, it plays a substantial role. Lifestyle is a factor as well: In a busy society, there's less time to focus on meal planning and preparation and more reliance on convenient, high-calorie, low-nutrient foods. The Paleo diet takes out the "sad" and centers our dietary focus on natural, unprocessed foods with high nutritional value.

Everything You Can Enjoy on Paleo

We've talked about everything you *cannot* have on the Paleo diet, but we haven't mentioned everything you *can* enjoy! When you begin to cook with fresh ingredients, your taste buds will awaken. Part of embracing Paleo is allowing yourself to experiment and find new ingredients to love. The Paleo diet can be so much more than its reputation of humdrum grilled chicken and steamed vegetables. It is a chance to learn healthy alternatives and easy swaps that can naturally become part of your daily eating. Instead of eating trans-fat-heavy French fries from the drive-through, you can try homemade Truffle Parsnip Fries (page 58), roasted in a pan in heart-healthy avocado oil. Instead of processed chocolate peanut butter cups, make homemade Almond Butter Cups (page 144). Paleo isn't about giving things up—it's about choosing better ingredients.

SO MANY FOODS TO ENJOY!

When we think of Paleo-friendly foods, we can break it down into five main categories: whole fruits and vegetables, nuts and seeds, healthy fats, lean proteins, and natural sweeteners. When deciding if a food is Paleo-compliant, check the ingredients for non-Paleo-friendly ingredients like processed sugars, soy, dairy, and preservatives. The foundation of a Paleo diet includes the following:

Whole fruits and vegetables—These are full of vitamins and minerals. Berries offer a high fiber content and antioxidant properties. Strawberries and blueberries both contain anthocyanins, which are known to support heart health. Citrus fruits are high in vitamin C, which supports the immune system, and they also have a low glycemic index, making them a sweet treat that won't spike your blood sugar. Spinach has a high iron and calcium content, making it a great addition to plant-based smoothies. Sweet potatoes are a staple in the Paleo diet—loaded with vitamins A and C and potassium, they are a great noninflammatory alternative to regular potatoes.

Nuts and seeds—These are greatly underrepresented in the Standard American Diet. While they make a great and filling snack on their own, they can also be toasted and added to a dish for added flavor and nutritional benefit. Nuts and seeds are loaded with healthy fats, protein, and fiber. Try adding toasted sunflower seeds to your next salad for extra nutrition and added crunch.

Healthy fats—Not all fats are created equal. Our body needs fat to survive, but we need to choose fats that promote heart and brain health. Trans fats, like those found in processed foods and prepackaged desserts, and saturated fats found in butter, red meat, and dairy, increase low-density lipoprotein (LDL) cholesterol levels in the body. LDL cholesterol can build up on the walls of the arteries, clogging them and increasing your risk of heart disease. Replacing saturated fats with unsaturated fats—like those found in olive oil, avocados, almonds, and salmon—actually lowers your risk of heart disease and stroke.

Lean proteins—Like fats, not all proteins are created equal either. Protein is an important part of the Paleo diet—but pay attention to the source. Organic, grass-fed meat sources tend to have lower overall fat. We recommend choosing antibiotic-free, organic chicken. When looking for seafood, wild-caught options tend to be slightly lower in saturated fat.

Natural sweeteners—We don't expect you to give up sweets completely! The Paleo diet is a lifestyle change—the changes you make should be ones you can maintain over the long time. Luckily, there are plenty of Paleo-friendly natural sweeteners, such as honey, maple syrup, coconut sugar, and fruit. In many recipes, a natural sweetener can be used as a 1:1 substitution. Try using coconut sugar in place of cane sugar in your next recipe or using maple syrup instead of brown sugar to sweeten a sauce.

The Paleo diet doesn't focus on what you cannot enjoy, but rather on easy adjustments you can make to your current diet that support your health without turning your world upside down. As you begin to experiment with recipes, you'll develop new ways to integrate healthy ingredients into your everyday cooking.

Ingredients That Aren't Considered Paleo

———————— ✕ ————————

While there is a diverse range of foods that are considered Paleo, there are a few categories that need to be avoided, primarily due to the inflammatory responses they can create in the body. We'll focus on grains, legumes, dairy, and processed sugars.

- *Grains and legumes* - Grains include ingredients like corn, oats, rice, wheat, and barley, while legumes include the pea family, such as lima beans, soybeans, peanuts, and chickpeas. Both grains and legumes have proteins called prolamins, which can play an important role in what is called "leaky gut syndrome." Prolamins can cause disruptions in the gut barrier, initiating an immune response within the intestinal layer and disrupting the balance of natural gut bacteria.

- *Dairy* - For many people, dairy is the hardest category to eliminate. When we are young, our pancreas produces lactase, the enzyme responsible for breaking down lactose, but in many people, this production stops around the age of two—worldwide, over 60 percent of adults are unable to digest lactose. When we cannot break down lactose, we experience inflammation.

- *Processed sugars* - Consuming too much sugar, no matter the source, can be dangerous for our health. Processed or refined sugars (such as high-fructose corn syrup) pose an even greater risk and have been linked to heart disease, liver disease, increased inflammation, and other complications.

GO CUISINE CRAZY

How often do you get bored of eating the same thing day in and day out? It is easy for us to fall into a routine with food, and often that routine is not the healthiest. Eating for convenience rarely correlates with eating for nutrition, due to the widespread availability of unhealthy options. While the Standard American Diet is far from Paleo, exploring new cuisines is a great way to mix it up a bit. There are many other cuisines from around the world that are naturally Paleo or can be easily modified to be Paleo-friendly.

Mediterranean-inspired food—The Mediterranean diet and the Paleo diet have many similarities and a few notable differences. The Mediterranean diet is a whole-food diet that relies on moderation instead of restriction. Like the Paleo diet, it focuses on fresh fruits and vegetables, nuts and seeds, and lean proteins. The main difference is that the Mediterranean diet permits grains, legumes, and dairy in moderation. Greek cuisine specifically is one of the most naturally Paleo-friendly cuisines. Try Baba Ghanoush (page 53) or Mediterranean-Style Steak Salad (page 77) to see how we create Mediterranean-inspired dishes that are Paleo-friendly.

Italian-inspired food—Italian food may not seem Paleo-friendly, with lots of pasta, carbs, and cream. Pasta certainly isn't Paleo-compliant, but there are many ways to design dishes around it. Spiralized vegetables are a great alternative to traditional pasta, and you can serve pasta sauces over sautéed vegetables instead. For instance, Chicken Puttanesca (page 111) can be served over zucchini noodles ("zoodles") or a medley of vegetables like squash, carrots, and spinach.

Indian-inspired food—Many Indian dishes are inherently Paleo, and many others are easy to make Paleo-friendly. Many dishes can be prepared with full-fat coconut milk rather than cream or yogurt, such as Tandoori-Style Chicken (page 104). Indian dishes are typically served with rice, but rice can be easily replaced by Cauliflower "Rice" (page 54) or other vegetables.

Korean-inspired food—The most Paleo-friendly component of the Standard American Diet may be barbecued or grilled meats—but American-style barbecue often relies on sugar-filled sauces or starch-filled sides. Korean cuisine also features grilled meats, but the sides are often vegetable-based.

Try pairing lean bulgogi (marinated grilled beef) with kimchi (fermented cabbage) for a protein-packed, gut-healthy meal.

Thai-inspired food—If you have access to fresh herbs and spices like ginger, lemongrass, mint, turmeric, and Thai basil, I encourage you to explore Thai cuisine. Many Thai recipes are served with rice, but again, you can easily substitute Cauliflower "Rice" (page 54). Many Thai curries are built around lean proteins, vegetables, and coconut milk, making them a fairly simple and very flavorful Paleo-friendly option to cook at home.

As you embrace the Paleo diet, it is our hope that you will try new ingredients, techniques, and recipes to incorporate into your daily cooking. One of the best ways to do this is to educate yourself about food that you may not have grown up eating. Don't be afraid to experiment and get creative with your food.

Talk to Your Doctor

--- × ---

While Paleo has become a popular diet in recent years, it may not be appropriate for everyone. Following a Paleo diet may be a stark shift in the way you eat, so it is important to speak with your doctor before you make such a significant lifestyle change. Paleo is a high-protein, low-carbohydrate diet. For those with kidney concerns, this may not be the best choice. Your doctor will be able to assess your current health situation and determine whether the Paleo diet is right for you.

Second, what we eat is only part of the equation. Maintaining a Paleo diet is not a substitute for engaging daily in physical activity and exercise. Your doctor will be able to recommend a level of physical activity that suits your specific needs.

Lastly, it is also important to understand that a diet is only powerful for as long as you can maintain it. Paleo is not designed to be a short-term diet; it is meant to be a lifestyle change that you carry with you throughout your life.

Paleo Portioning Plates

The USDA-recommended food guidelines for portion and serving sizes have changed over the years. You may recall the food pyramid of the early 1990s, with the largest food group at the bottom of the pyramid being 6–11 recommended servings of "breads, cereals, rice, and pasta." The second-largest food groups on the pyramid were fruits and vegetables, then smaller sections for meat and dairy, and the smallest section for fat. The food guidelines were most recently updated in 2011 and rebranded to MyPlate. On the MyPlate guidelines, the largest portions are equal amounts of vegetables and grains. Protein and fruit are slightly smaller, and there is a small portion recommended for dairy. Fat appears nowhere in the 2011 guidelines.

If you were to draw a pyramid or plate for the Paleo diet, it would look significantly different from any of the USDA diagrams. The largest portion on a Paleo plate should be vegetables, followed by protein. A portion of healthy fats should be included in every meal and snack. Grains are eliminated completely. Let's break down each component on the Paleo plate and discuss its importance.

Vegetables make up the largest food group on a Paleo plate. They are filled with vitamins and minerals and naturally contain a source of complex carbohydrates, which provide energy. Starchy vegetables like sweet potatoes, butternut squash, and parsnips are higher in carbohydrates than leafy ones, so be aware of how often you are consuming them.

Lean proteins are the next largest food group on the Paleo diet. This includes wild-caught fish, grass-fed organic beef, and antibiotic-free and organic poultry. These foods provide the protein your body needs to build and repair tissue.

The remainder of the plate should be made up of healthy fats and fruits. Fat is essential for brain and body function, and fruits contain natural sugars and complex carbohydrates for added energy.

Paleo Plate Portioning

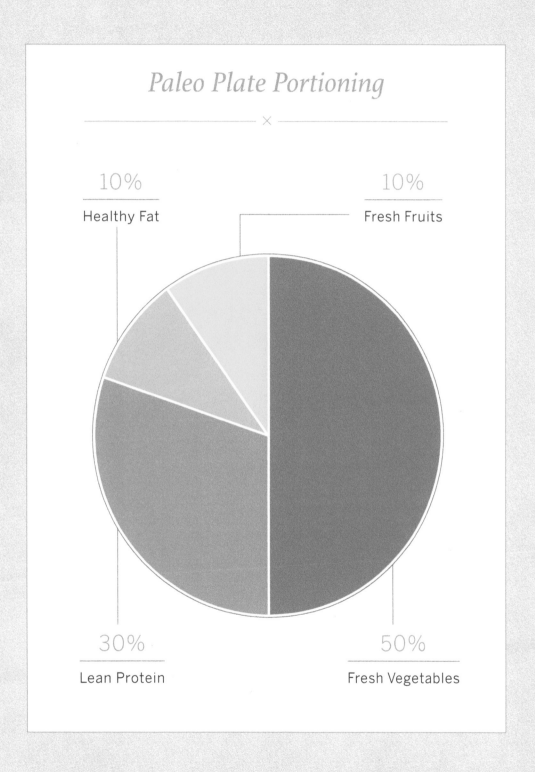

10%
Healthy Fat

10%
Fresh Fruits

30%
Lean Protein

50%
Fresh Vegetables

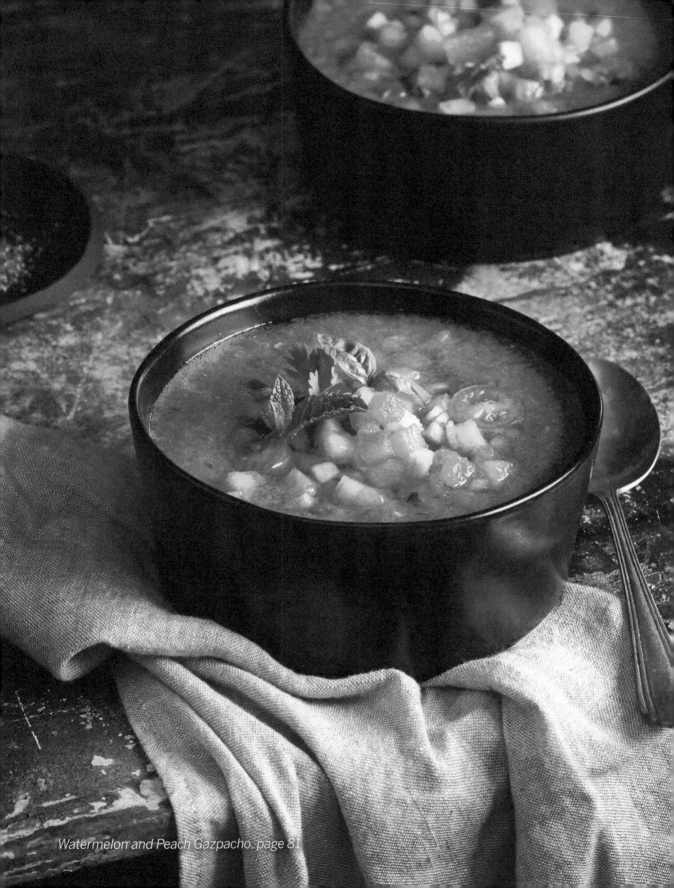

Watermelon and Peach Gazpacho, page 81

CHAPTER TWO

Cooking Paleo for Two

Cooking for two should be fun! Smaller-batch recipes allow you to get creative and be flexible with ingredients and techniques to prepare unique and flavorful dishes. In this chapter, we will include tips for shopping and cooking for two so that it can become second nature to you. We set you up for success with key ingredients to include in your pantry to make your transition to the Paleo diet a breeze.

Learning to Cook for Two

Maybe you're newlyweds. Maybe you're roommates balancing college or a job with a healthier lifestyle, or perhaps you're a single parent cooking for yourself and your child. So many of us are cooking for two, but many recipes are written for large families or groups. This book was written just for you.

Cooking for two is a great way to work together as a team toward a common goal. Depending on your experience with cooking, there may be a lot to learn about ingredients, techniques, and your own personal taste. As with any team, there are roles to be played, and you may surprise each other with your respective skills. If you're a parent, involve your child in the process by having them help wash the vegetables, scrape the bowls, and of course, be the official taste tester.

HOW IS IT DIFFERENT?

Cooking for two people requires a different approach, but your shopping habits don't have to change much. You can still take advantage of budget-saving bulk-buy opportunities for meat or produce, but instead of using everything at once, you'll break ingredients down into smaller batches for preparation and later use. Smaller recipes will also allow you to explore new ingredients and preparations that larger families may avoid. Buying lamb or wild-caught fish for six people can be cost-prohibitive, but if you are only serving two, it's suddenly affordable.

Whether you are feeding two or eight, planning meals is an essential part of establishing a weekly routine for a healthy diet. Keep it exciting by challenging yourself to try one new protein, vegetable, seasoning, or spice each week. While new ingredients are great, it's also always important to have few basic recipes to fall back on. These recipes should require minimal advanced prep, rely on staple ingredients, and be quick and easy to throw together without a mess.

Perhaps the most difficult part of the Paleo diet—or any healthy diet—is avoiding giving in to convenience foods. Our lives are busy, and if you don't plan for it, something will always get in the way of cooking. For that reason, this book focuses on quick and easy meals for those nights when the drive-through is a strong temptation.

OPPORTUNITIES FOR SHOPPING AND COOKING TOGETHER

Cooking is a team effort, and there are ways to divide prepping tasks so that each person contributes to the final product. There are five main components to successfully executing the Paleo diet:

1. Menu planning

2. Grocery shopping

3. Prepping

4. Cooking

5. Cleaning up

When cooking for two, both people can and should be involved. We encourage rotating tasks, so that each person has a turn in each position. We especially recommend this if one of you is typically "in charge" of meals—allowing yourselves to step out of your comfort zones is a great way to challenge yourselves and to make sure each person has agency.

If you're a parent and child, involve your child in the decision-making, cooking, and cleaning processes to whatever extent you are able. You may be surprised by what your child can do!

Tips for Cooking Two-gether

—————————————— ✕ ——————————————

Cooking together is a great team-building exercise, and no one person should pull all the weight. Take turns acting as the sous-chef—a professional chef's second in command. Sous-chefs prepare ingredients in a timely and organized way to set the chef up for success. Prep tasks typical for a sous-chef—like chopping, mincing, dicing, and blending—can usually be done either in advance or as the meal is being cooked.

Depending on the layout of your kitchen, you may want to set up two separate stations: one for preparation and one for cooking. This will keep your respective areas tidy and all the components consolidated. Once the prep is done, the prepper can move on to plating or cleaning. One of the biggest tips we can offer is to do dishes as you go. Keeping up with cleaning throughout the process will avoid a sink or counter full of dirty dishes to deal with later.

Planning Your Paleo Kitchen

Alexander Graham Bell once said, "Before anything else, preparation is the key to success"—and we couldn't agree more. Setting up your pantry, refrigerator, and kitchen with ingredients and tools that allow for Paleo-friendly cooking will make all the difference once you get going. Humans are creatures of habit and convenience, and we tend to gravitate toward what is ready, available, and easiest to access—so we have to make healthy food accessible and easy. If you don't have unhealthy foods at home, you won't be tempted to eat them. But if you stock your pantry and refrigerator with healthy and nutritious snacks and ingredients, you'll turn toward them when a craving hits. We'll go over key ingredients, including Paleo-friendly substitutes to keep on hand for recipes, as well as emergency snacks to keep sugar cravings at bay. We'll also cover a few key kitchen tools to make cooking easier.

FOODS TO HAVE ON HAND

Choosing healthy substitutes for non-Paleo-friendly ingredients is key to stocking a Paleo kitchen. There are three main areas to cover: the refrigerator, freezer, and pantry.

Refrigerator

- » Unsweetened almond milk and coconut milk (instead of milk)
- » Coconut oil (instead of butter)
- » Coconut aminos (instead of soy sauce)
- » Cashew cheese (instead of dairy cheese)
- » Fresh fruits and vegetables
- » Basic Vinaigrette (page 153) (for salads)
- » Guilt-Free Ranch Dressing (page 160) (for sandwiches and salads)

Freezer

- » Organic mixed frozen berries (for smoothies, pancakes, or waffles)
- » Almond Meal Sandwich Bread (page 121) (for sandwiches)
- » Frozen wild-caught salmon (for "emergency" dinners that can be quickly thawed when needed)

Pantry

- » Tapioca starch, almond meal and flour (natural and blanched), coconut flour, and arrowroot starch (instead of wheat-based flour)
- » Honey, maple syrup, and coconut sugar (instead of cane sugar)
- » Dried fruits, dry-roasted nuts, and all-natural protein bars (instead of junk food snacks)
- » Almond butter (instead of peanut butter, for smoothies, sandwiches, and snacks)
- » Nutritional yeast
- » Dried herbs and spices, such as sea salt, black pepper, red pepper flakes, garlic powder, onion powder, and Italian seasoning

Where to Shop for What

—————————— × ——————————

Stocking your pantry for Paleo cooking may feel overwhelming or a bit costly at first, but there are many ingredients you can buy in bulk that will last a long time once purchased. Bulk discount stores like Costco and Sam's Club often have ingredients that are great for Paleo cooking (though it's important to read through ingredient lists when shopping to ensure they don't contain preservatives or stabilizers). We'll divide pantry staples into the following categories: proteins, fruits and vegetables, flours, sweeteners, fats, and seasonings.

- Proteins - Choose grass-fed and grass-finished beef, organic and antibiotic-free chicken, pasture-raised pork, cage-free eggs, and wild-caught seafood. This is a place to spend—protein should be the same high quality as any other ingredients you use. If you have the storage space, we also recommend contacting a local farm to purchase a quarter or half of a cow, as many will butcher it and separate the cuts of meat for you.

- Fruits and Vegetables - Choose organic fruits and vegetables whenever possible. We like to shop for produce at Whole Foods, Sprouts, and, whenever possible, our local farmers' market.

- Flours - Many recipes in this book rely on almond flour or almond meal. There are two types of almond meal: natural and blanched. Natural almond meal is less expensive and works in most recipes. The recipes in this book also use coconut flour and tapioca starch. Often, your best option

for specialty flours is the Internet—look for bulk deals on Amazon or Nuts.com.

- *Sweeteners* - We recommend buying local honey from the farmers market whenever possible. Invest in high-quality honey and maple syrup from small-batch distributors. Look for dried fruit online, from retailers like Nuts.com or Mount Hope Wholesale.

- *Fats* - You may have used vegetable oils like canola or corn oil in the past, but for Paleo cooking, you'll switch to extra-virgin olive oil, avocado oil, and coconut oil. Bulk stores nowadays generally have large bottles of all of these. Cooking oils won't spoil quickly, so get a big bottle and use it for a long time.

- *Seasonings* - Fresh herbs can elevate flavors when cooking and many (like basil, rosemary, chives, and mint) can be grown indoors quite easily. Dried herbs and spices will keep for quite some time, so for common ingredients, you may want to purchase a large container from a bulk foods store.

HANDY KITCHEN EQUIPMENT AND TOOLS

Having the right tools on hand will make it easy to get comfortable with cooking Paleo. Here are some essentials we recommend as you're starting out.

Knives—You'll use knives more than anything else in your kitchen, so it's important to invest in a couple of high-quality knives for chopping, dicing, and slicing. You'll need a small paring knife for smaller cuts, as well as a larger chef's knife. We also recommend a high-quality bread knife for slicing homemade Almond Meal Sandwich Bread (page 121).

Cutting board—We recommend at least two cutting boards: one for produce and one for meat.

Pots and pans—For the recipes in this book, you'll need a small saucepan and large pot with lids and small and large nonstick sauté pans. You'll also need a standard-size loaf pan (8½-by-4½-inch or 9-by-5-inch), a 9-by-13-inch baking dish, a 12-cup muffin tin, a 9-inch pie dish, and an 8- or 9-inch square baking dish.

Utensils—You may already have a few cooking utensils. Make sure you have wooden mixing spoons, metal and silicone spatulas, a whisk, and a ladle, as well as a can opener and a vegetable peeler.

Measuring cups and spoons—A full set of measuring spoons should cover amounts from ⅛ teaspoon to 1 tablespoon, and dry measuring cups should go from ¼ cup to 1 cup. We also recommend a 2-cup glass liquid measuring cup.

Rolling pin—In this book, we use a rolling pin to make Tortilla Chips (page 125) and Everything Seed Crackers (page 55). We recommend either a marble or wood rolling pin, rather than plastic. Wood rolling pins are lighter, but they are harder to clean than marble.

Blender—Choose a blender that meets your needs and fits your budget. An upright blender (like a Ninja or Vitamix) will easily make supersmooth break-fast smoothies, but you can also get by with an affordable handheld immersion blender, which is perfect for making sauces and dressings and requires much less cleanup.

Mixer—As with the blender, choose a mixer that suits your needs. This can range from a handheld electric mixer to a Kitchen-Aid stand mixer, depending on your budget, but know that either will work well for the recipes in this book.

Oven mitts and kitchen towels—Invest in a high-quality oven mitt (or two) to protect your hands when removing hot dishes or trays from the oven. We also recommend placing a damp kitchen towel beneath your cutting board to prevent it from sliding on the counter.

For the recipes in this book, there are a few other kitchen tools that are nice to have, but not necessary. Some dishes can be prepared with less hands-on cooking time by using either a slow cooker or electric pressure cooker (like the Instant Pot), but they can also be prepared using other methods if you don't have either. An ice cream maker will speed up the process for the Pineapple Sorbet (page 141) and Vanilla Bean Ice Cream (page 135), but they can also be made by hand using only your freezer. Once you have stocked your kitchen with the essential tools, you'll be ready to prepare virtually any recipe in this book and beyond.

The Recipes

The recipes in this book are separated into eight chapters—Breakfast, Snacks and Sides, Salads, Soups and Sandwiches, Mains, Breads and Baked Goods, Desserts, and Staples, Sauces and Dressings—to provide you Paleo-friendly options to meet any craving head-on. If you are newer to cooking, we recommend starting with simpler "5-Ingredient" and "One-Pot" recipes (pages 172 and 174–175) and working your way up to more advanced dishes.

When we chose the recipes for this cookbook, we wanted to include a wide variety of flavor profiles to introduce you to new seasonings and ingredients you may not have tried before. We also included a number of vegetarian dishes for those following a plant-based Paleo diet.

We included certain recipes with seasons, holidays, and seasonal vegetables in mind, like Bread Crumb Dressing (page 131) for Thanksgiving or refreshing Watermelon and Peach Gazpacho (page 81) for warm summer days. With that said, all of these recipes can be enjoyed year-round. We hope that the variety will make you excited about your meals and keep you happy, healthy, and Paleo-friendly.

HOW TO SCALE WHEN COOKING FOR TWO

While this book is designed around recipes to feed two people, there will be times when you want to feed a larger group but stay Paleo-compliant. Look for recipes with "Scale It Up" tips, which include advice to scale up entire recipes or prep larger amounts for quicker cooking later on. Preparing certain frequently used Paleo basics in advance, like Breakfast Sausage (page 38) and Almond Meal Sandwich Bread (page 121), will help make cooking faster.

Storage is as important as prep, especially when you're freezing a meal, and we'll provide freezing instructions to ensure long-term freshness.

When you double a recipe for baking, you generally do so by doubling each individual ingredient. With cooking, this is not always the case. For instance, when doubling a recipe that involves marinating meat, you'll double the amount of meat but can use the same amount of marinade. When it's relevant, we'll provide specific instructions for scaling up individual recipes to ensure you are set up for fool-proof cooking.

CARB COUNTS AND NUTRITIONAL INFORMATION

While these recipes all use Paleo-friendly ingredients and guidelines, there are still some ingredients to look out for, especially if you're pursuing a low-carbohydrate diet. You may wish to avoid recipes that use tapioca starch or arrowroot starch, which are both higher in carbohydrates than seed- and nut-based flours like almond meal and coconut flour. Likewise, sweet potatoes, parsnips, and other starchy vegetables are higher in carbohydrates than leafy green vegetables.

No matter your goals with Paleo, it is important to track your nutritional intake. If you're looking to lose weight, you may want to err on the side of lower carbohydrate intake, limiting starchy flours and vegetables and focusing instead on lean protein and healthy fats like salmon and avocado. If you are looking to improve energy and strength, you may want to follow a slightly higher-carbohydrate base. Take note of the nutrition information after the recipe and use the labels discussed in the next section to quickly identify the best recipes for your needs.

LABELS

All the recipes in this book are designed to fall into subcategories to make it easy for you to find recipes that work for you. The labels used in the recipes are:

One-Pot—Dishes that are designed so that all ingredients can be prepared in a single pot or dish. Once cooked, the dish can be served in a single bowl as a complete meal. One-pot meals are great for small kitchens, as they require fewer dishes and less preparation and generally make less of a mess.

30 Minutes and **5-Ingredient**—Great recipes for last-minute emergency meals, quick to prepare and made with ingredients that you likely already have on hand. Both of these are what they sound like—recipes labeled "30 Minutes" can be prepared in under half an hour. Recipes labeled "5-Ingredient" use five ingredients or less, not counting salt, black pepper, olive oil, and water.

Vegetarian—Many people assume that it's impossible to be vegetarian on the Paleo diet, but this is not the case. There are many Paleo-friendly sources of plant-based protein, and we have included several healthy vegetarian recipes in this book.

Diabetes-Friendly—These recipes have especially low (or no) carbohydrates, for those who have chosen the Paleo diet with a focus on keeping insulin levels stable. While Paleo is already a low-carb and high-protein diet, we have highlighted the recipes that are truly low-carb and will work for those who are cooking with diabetes in mind.

Low-Carb—These recipes are great for people who may be embracing the Paleo diet as a way to lose weight. In recipes labeled "Low-Carb" in this book, carbohydrates make up less than 8 percent of the total nutritional content. For instance, a recipe that makes 100 grams would have to have 8 or fewer grams of carbohydrates.

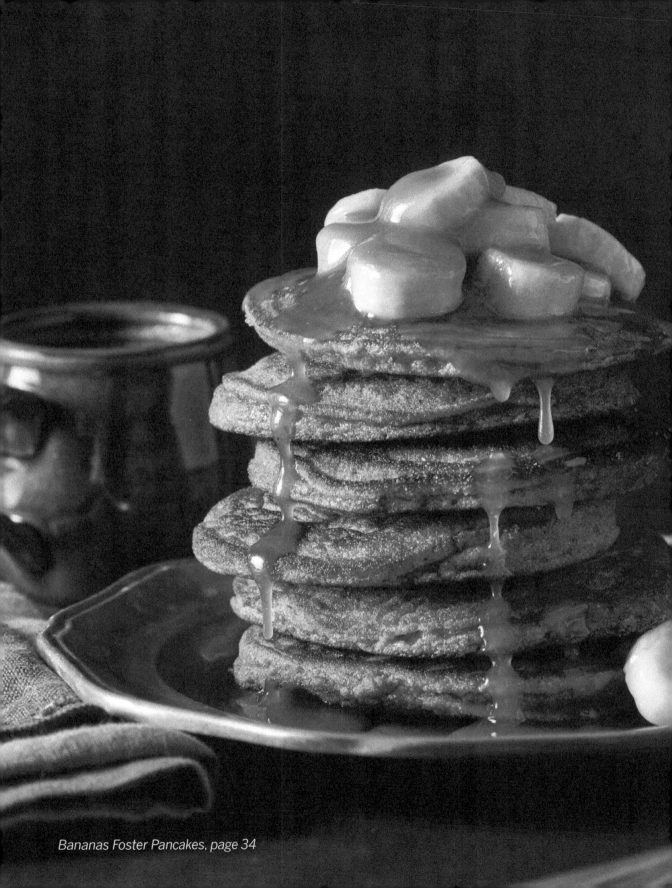

Bananas Foster Pancakes, page 34

CHAPTER THREE

Breakfast

— ◇ —

We all know that breakfast "breaks your fast," making it the most important meal that jump-starts your metabolism for the day. A Paleo-friendly breakfast needs a balance of protein, healthy fats, and slow-burning carbohydrates. In the Standard American Diet, breakfast often consists of fast-burning carbohydrates, like sugary cereals or pancakes without sufficient nutrients, leaving you hungry and depleted of energy after a short time.

In this chapter, we introduce a variety of sweet and savory breakfast options to kick-start your metabolism and keep you satisfied until lunchtime. Most of these Paleo-friendly breakfasts are high in protein, including quick and easy on-the-go breakfasts like smoothies as well as more complex dishes for a luxurious weekend brunch, like Baked French Toast (page 28).

Avocado Baked Eggs

» Vegetarian, Low-Carb, Diabetes-Friendly, 30 Minutes

» Serves 2

» Prep time: 5 minutes
Cook time: 10 minutes

This quick, easy, and super flavorful breakfast recipe is great for a busy weekday morning. The prep work is minimal, and the dish can bake while you are getting ready for work. Eggs offer protein to counterbalance the healthy fat of the avocados, ensuring that this dish fills you up without weighing you down.

3 large avocados

Pinch sea salt

Pinch freshly ground
black pepper

6 large eggs

2 limes, juiced

¼ cup chopped cilantro

¼ cup sliced scallions

¼ teaspoon red
pepper flakes

1. Preheat the oven to 425°F.

2. Cut each avocado in half lengthwise and remove and discard the pit. Using a spoon, gently widen the well in the center of each avocado to allow room for an egg.

3. Season the avocados with salt and pepper and place them in an 8-by-8-inch baking dish. Crack an egg into the center of each avocado.

4. Bake the avocados and eggs for 8 to 12 minutes, until the egg whites are fully set. Remove the avocados from the oven and garnish them with the lime juice, cilantro, scallions, and red pepper flakes. Serve immediately.

Make It Easier: Don't like a runny yolk? Pre-scramble your eggs before pouring them into the avocados and bake for the same amount of time. Both the egg white and yolk will cook through, but you won't risk overcooking the avocado.

PER SERVING: *Calories: 776; Total fat: 60g; Sodium: 303mg; Carbohydrates: 41g; Fiber: 26g; Protein: 29g; Iron: 4mg*

Baked French Toast

» Vegetarian   » Serves 2   » Prep time: 15 minutes
Cook time: 30 minutes

French toast can be prepared on the stovetop or in the oven. In this recipe, we use the oven because it's hands-off. If you choose to cook your French toast in a sauté pan on the stovetop, make sure the heat is low so that it doesn't burn the toast. French toast should typically only be flipped one time—a handy rule of thumb is that if the bread does not release easily from the pan, it is not ready to flip.

6 large eggs

1½ cups full-fat coconut milk

¼ cup sweetener of your choice (such as coconut sugar, maple syrup, or honey)

Zest of 1 orange

1 teaspoon cinnamon

¼ teaspoon ground nutmeg

½ teaspoon sea salt

4 thick slices day-old Almond Meal Sandwich Bread (page 121)

1 cup coarsely chopped pecans (optional)

1 cup maple syrup, for serving

¼ cup raisins (optional)

1. Preheat the oven to 375°F

2. In a medium bowl, whisk the eggs until they are pale yellow. Then, whisk in the coconut milk, your sweetener of choice, orange zest, cinnamon, nutmeg, and salt.

3. Working in batches, dip the bread slices into the egg mixture to coat, pressing down gently to submerge. Let the bread soak for 5 minutes, then flip it and soak the second side for 5 minutes.

4. Lay the soaked bread slices in an 8-by-8-inch baking dish (some overlapping is okay). Bake, uncovered, for 15 minutes.

5. Remove the dish from the oven and sprinkle it with pecans (if using). Return the dish to the oven and bake for an additional 10 minutes. If not using pecans, simply leave the dish in the oven for 10 additional minutes.

6. While the French toast bakes, make the syrup. In a small saucepan over medium-low heat, combine the maple syrup and raisins (if using). Bring the mixture to a rapid boil, stirring often, then reduce the heat to low and simmer for 5 to 10 minutes. Remove from the heat and set aside.

7. Remove the French toast from the oven and serve it with the syrup.

Scale It Up: This recipe can easily be doubled or tripled to feed a crowd or to have leftovers. To store French toast, let it cool at room temperature and wrap each slice in plastic wrap. Place the slices in a freezer-safe resealable bag. Reheat the slices in the oven or toaster oven at 375°F for 8 to 10 minutes, until heated through.

PER SERVING: *Calories: 1485; Total fat: 86g; Sodium: 1133mg; Carbohydrates: 153g; Fiber: 6g; Protein: 38g; Iron: 12mg*

Wild Mushroom Gravy

» One-Pot, Vegetarian   » Serves 2   » Prep time: 15 minutes
Cook time: 20 minutes

This recipe can be made with any type of wild mushrooms, from mild white button mushrooms to bold shiitakes. Mushrooms are often used in place of meat as a vegetarian substitute due to the rich umami flavor they offer once cooked (umami is a Japanese word that means "a pleasant savory taste"). We like to use a blend of shiitake, cremini, and porcini mushrooms.

2 tablespoons olive oil

1 shallot, minced

1 cup thinly sliced
   wild mushrooms of
   your choice

2 garlic cloves, minced

1 cup full-fat coconut milk

1 tablespoon plus
   1½ teaspoons tapioca
   flour

1 teaspoon chopped
   fresh sage

1 teaspoon chopped
   fresh thyme

½ teaspoon sea salt

¼ teaspoon freshly ground
   black pepper

1. Heat the olive oil in a large sauté pan over medium heat. Once hot, add the shallot and cook until translucent and slightly browned, 2 to 3 minutes.

2. Add the mushrooms to the sauté pan and cook, stirring frequently, for 8 to 10 minutes, allowing the mushrooms to release their juices and begin to brown. Add the garlic and sauté for 1 minute.

3. In a small mixing bowl, combine the coconut milk and tapioca flour and whisk until combined. Add this mixture to the sauté pan and simmer for 5 minutes, or until the gravy reaches your desired consistency.

4. Add the sage, thyme, salt, and pepper and stir to incorporate. Remove from the heat.

5. Store the gravy in an airtight container in the refrigerator for up to 4 days or freeze it in a freezer-safe resealable bag for up to 2 months. To reheat the gravy, warm it on the stovetop, adding in 2 tablespoons water per serving.

Make It Easier: To save time, you can use dried herbs. A general rule of thumb when substituting dry herbs for fresh herbs is to reduce the amount by half, since dried herbs are more concentrated in flavor.

PER SERVING: *Calories: 385; Total fat: 38g; Sodium: 309mg; Carbohydrates: 13g; Fiber: 1g; Protein: 4g; Iron: 4mg*

Avocado Toast (on Sweet Potatoes!)

» Vegetarian, 30 Minutes   » Serves 2   » Prep time: 10 minutes
Cook time: 20 minutes

Many of us are familiar with sweet potatoes with orange flesh, but there are several kinds of sweet potatoes, including ones with purple and white flesh. Any type of sweet potato can be used in this recipe—all varieties are high in fiber, vitamins, and antioxidants. Consider using a mix of different sweet potatoes for a colorful plate.

2 medium sweet potatoes

1 tablespoon olive oil

1 teaspoon sea salt

¼ teaspoon freshly ground black pepper

2 avocados

Zest and juice of 1 lime

2 tablespoons sliced scallions, for garnish

1 teaspoon crushed red pepper flakes, for garnish (optional)

6 cherry tomatoes, quartered, for garnish

2 tablespoons sprouts, for garnish

1. Preheat the oven to 400°F and line a baking sheet with aluminum foil.

2. Wash and scrub the sweet potatoes and remove any tough ends or roots. Slice the potatoes lengthwise into ½-inch-thick slices. Discard the end pieces or reserve them for another dish.

3. Lay the sweet potato slices on the baking sheet, drizzle them with olive oil, and season them with salt and pepper. Bake for 10 minutes on each side, until they can be easily pierced with a fork.

4. While the sweet potatoes bake, make the avocado mash. Halve the avocados and discard the pits. Using a spoon, gently scrape the flesh into a bowl and mash with a fork. Add the lime juice and zest and stir to combine.

5. Once the sweet potatoes are ready, remove them from the oven and transfer them to plates. Top them with avocado mash and garnish with scallions, red pepper flakes (if using), cherry tomatoes, and sprouts. Serve immediately.

Ingredient Swaps: The avocado mash can also be served on toasted Almond Meal Sandwich Bread (page 121) instead of sweet potato slices.

PER SERVING: *Calories: 558; Total fat: 38g; Sodium: 664mg; Carbohydrates: 55g; Fiber: 22g; Protein: 10g; Iron: 2mg*

Steak and Sweet Potato Breakfast Hash

» 30 Minutes

» Serves 2

» Prep time: 5 minutes, plus 1 hour to marinate
Cook time: 25 minutes

This breakfast hash is one of the most versatile dishes in this cookbook—you can substitute any protein or vegetable. Use dinner leftovers, add spices, and roast and in minutes you'll have a delicious and nutritious breakfast. Try topping the hash with eggs over-easy for extra protein. If making this dish fresh, we recommend marinating the steak the night before so you can cook it quickly the next morning.

1 pound steak (sirloin, flank, or flat iron)

1 tablespoon red wine vinegar

1 teaspoon red pepper flakes

2 teaspoons sea salt, divided

1 teaspoon paprika

1 teaspoon dried oregano

½ teaspoon freshly ground black pepper

½ teaspoon cayenne pepper

¼ teaspoon ground cinnamon

4 tablespoons olive oil, divided

2 medium sweet potatoes, peeled and cut into ½-inch cubes

1. Preheat the oven to 400°F and line a baking sheet with aluminum foil.

2. Prepare the steak to marinate. Cut the steak into bite-size pieces and transfer it to a medium bowl. Add the vinegar, red pepper flakes, 1 teaspoon salt, paprika, oregano, black pepper, cayenne pepper, and cinnamon. Mix well and let the steak marinate for at least 1 hour, or up to 24 hours.

3. Heat 2 tablespoons olive oil in a large nonstick sauté pan over medium-high heat. Once the oil is shimmering, add the marinated steak and cook for 4 minutes, flipping halfway through to ensure even searing. Remove the steak from the pan and set aside. It won't be cooked through, but it will finish cooking in the oven.

4. In a large bowl, toss the sweet potatoes, bell pepper, and onion with the remaining 2 tablespoons olive oil. Transfer the mixture to the baking sheet. Season with the remaining 1 teaspoon sea salt and roast for 20 minutes, or until the sweet potatoes are tender.

5. Remove the baking sheet from the oven, add the steak, and return it to the oven for 5 more minutes.

1 small bell pepper, diced

1 small red onion, diced

¼ cup freshly chopped parsley, for garnish

1 tablespoon freshly chopped cilantro, for garnish

6. Garnish with chopped parsley and cilantro and serve immediately.

Make It Easier: Save time by using leftovers. If you have even a little bit of dinner left at night, before you toss it, think about adding it to breakfast in the morning. Precooked vegetables and proteins make this dish quick and easy to throw together.

PER SERVING: *Calories: 761; Total fat: 46g; Sodium: 1366mg; Carbohydrates: 34g; Fiber: 7g; Protein: 51g; Iron: 6mg*

Bananas Foster Pancakes

» Vegetarian

» Serves 4

» Prep time: 1 hour
Cook time: 20 minutes

Bananas Foster is a dessert that was created in New Orleans. Traditionally, bananas are cooked in brown sugar and butter and then doused with rum. We changed up the ingredients to make this dish Paleo-friendly, but the essence shines through. The sauce can be used for other desserts or drizzled over Vanilla Bean Ice Cream (page 135). The pancake batter should rest for 30 minutes to 1 hour before cooking, so use that time to make the sauce.

For the pancakes

6 large eggs
¼ cup honey
1 teaspoon vanilla extract
¾ cup almond meal
¼ cup coconut flour
1 tablespoon ground flax-
  seed (or flax meal)
½ teaspoon baking soda
1 tablespoon ground
  cinnamon
¼ teaspoon sea salt
Olive oil cooking spray, for
  greasing the pan

For the sauce

4 bananas
¼ cup olive oil
¼ cup coconut sugar
1 cup honey
1 teaspoon vanilla extract
½ teaspoon
  almond extract
1 cup full-fat coconut milk
½ teaspoon sea salt

1. **Make the pancake batter.** Add the eggs, honey, and vanilla to the bowl of a stand mixer with the paddle attachment. Mix on medium speed to combine.

2. In a small mixing bowl, combine the almond meal, coconut flour, flaxseed, baking soda, cinnamon, and salt. Stir the mixture gently to combine.

3. Turn the mixer speed to low and slowly add the dry ingredients. Mix for 3 minutes, or until fully combined. Let the batter rest in the refrigerator for 30 minutes to 1 hour while you make the sauce.

4. **Make the sauce.** Slice the bananas into ½-inch rounds and set aside. Heat the olive oil and coconut sugar in a small saucepan over medium-low heat until it begins to bubble. Add the honey, vanilla, almond extract, and coconut milk and simmer for 7 to 10 minutes. Fold in the bananas and salt. Set aside to cool slightly.

5. Coat a medium nonstick sauté pan with olive oil cooking spray and heat on the lowest temperature. Drop 2 tablespoons of pancake batter at a time into the pan, spacing the pancakes about an inch apart. Cook on one side for 2 minutes, or until the center starts to bubble. Then flip the pancakes and cook for an additional 2 minutes on the other side.

6. Transfer finished pancakes to a cooling rack. Serve the finished pancakes hot, drizzled with the sauce.

Make It Easier: The pancake batter can be made ahead and refrigerated for up to 72 hours. Make the batter the night before to make breakfast prep a breeze on weekend mornings.

PER SERVING: *Calories: 946; Total fat: 41g; Sodium: 510mg; Carbohydrates: 139g; Fiber: 9g; Protein: 18g; Iron: 6mg*

Chicken, Mushroom, and Baby Kale Frittata

» Low-Carb, Diabetes-Friendly

» Serves 2

» Prep time: 15 minutes
Cook time: 30 minutes

The word "frittata," which comes from Italy, is used to describe an egg dish cooked in a pan with butter or oil. It is sometimes referred to as a "crustless quiche." Frittatas are very versatile, as they can be made with almost any proteins and vegetables, making them a great option for using up leftovers. Add some fresh spinach or kale and herbs to your dinner leftovers and you have a hearty and healthy breakfast in a snap.

6 eggs

½ cup full-fat coconut milk

1 tablespoon olive oil

1 shallot, diced

1 tablespoon garlic, minced

4 ounces sliced mushrooms (button, baby bella, shiitake, or cremini)

½ teaspoon sea salt

¼ teaspoon freshly ground black pepper

6 ounces cooked chicken breast, diced

1 cup coarsely chopped baby kale

Olive oil cooking spray, for greasing the pan (optional)

1. Preheat the oven to 350°F.

2. In a small bowl, whisk together the eggs and coconut milk and set aside.

3. Heat the olive oil in a medium sauté pan over medium heat. Add the shallot, garlic, mushrooms, salt, and pepper and sauté until the shallot are tender and translucent. Add the chicken breast and baby kale and cook for 1 minute.

4. Fold the vegetable and protein mixture into the egg mixture and transfer it to an 8-by-8-inch nonstick baking dish (coat generously with olive oil cooking spray, if necessary).

5. Bake the frittata for 30 minutes, or until the center is fully set. Serve hot.

Make It Easier: This dish is a great use of leftover chicken from yesterday's dinner. Save any leftover chicken or cook an extra piece to use in your breakfast the next day. Experiment with adding in leftover vegetables, like broccoli, squash, zucchini, or peppers.

PER SERVING: *Calories: 552; Total fat: 36g; Sodium: 581mg; Carbohydrates: 7g; Fiber: 1g; Protein: 49g; Iron: 6mg*

Almond Butter and Blueberry Smoothie

» 30 Minutes, Vegetarian,
5-Ingredient

» Serves 2

» Prep time: 5 minutes

This recipe puts two superfoods—blueberries and spinach—at center stage. Both are filled with vitamins and minerals to promote bone, skin, heart, hair, mental, and digestive health. The subtle sweetness and richness of almond butter pairs perfectly with the tart blueberries, making this smoothie dessert-worthy but still a healthy breakfast.

2 cups frozen blueberries

1 cup raw baby spinach

2 tablespoons
almond butter

1 tablespoon maple syrup

1/8 teaspoon sea salt

1 cup unsweetened
almond milk

Combine the blueberries, spinach, almond butter, maple syrup, salt, and almond milk in a blender. Blend on medium speed for 2 minutes, pausing to mix with a spoon if necessary. Pour into 2 glasses and serve immediately.

Make It Easier: To make this smoothie cost-effective, purchase a large bag of frozen wild blueberries from a bulk store like Costco or Sam's Club. Alternatively, freeze leftover fresh berries that are on the way out.

PER SERVING: *Calories: 260; Total fat: 15g; Sodium: 320mg; Carbohydrates: 30g; Fiber: 5g; Protein: 5g; Iron: 1mg*

Breakfast Sausage

» One-Pot, 30 Minutes

» Makes 4
(4-ounce) patties

» Prep time: 5 minutes
Cook time: 10 minutes

This Breakfast Sausage recipe will fill your kitchen with the aromas of sage and maple syrup. It's a staple that highlights flavors we crave while eliminating processed sugars, nitrates, binders, and other ingredients harmful to our health. Keep extra batches of this recipe on hand to use in other dishes, such as Breakfast Sausage-Stuffed Peppers (page 41).

1 pound ground pork
2 tablespoons maple syrup
2 teaspoons dried sage
1 tablespoon garlic powder
1 tablespoon onion powder
1 tablespoon sea salt
2 teaspoons freshly ground
  black pepper
½ teaspoon red
  pepper flakes
2 teaspoons olive oil
  (for cooking)

1. Add the pork, maple syrup, sage, garlic powder, onion powder, salt, pepper, and red pepper to the bowl of a stand mixer fitted with the paddle attachment. Mix on low speed for 3 minutes. If using this recipe as loose sausage, you can stop here and save it for cooking.

2. If making patties, use a scale or ¼-cup measuring cup to divide the meat into four 2-ounce portions. Shape the portions into 2-inch patties. If using later, you can freeze raw sausage patties for up to 2 months.

3. Heat the olive oil in a nonstick sauté pan over medium heat. Add the sausage patties to the pan and cook for 4 minutes on each side, or until cooked through. Serve hot.

Scale It Up: This Breakfast Sausage is extremely versatile and is a great staple to keep on hand. Double or triple this recipe to have it ready for frittatas, hashes, or a delicious breakfast side for your next gathering.

PER SERVING: *Calories: 198; Total fat: 7g; Sodium: 952mg; Carbohydrates: 10g; Fiber: 1g; Protein: 25g; Iron: 2mg*

Chocolate-Covered Strawberry Protein Bars

» 30 Minutes, Vegetarian   » Makes 9 bars   » Prep time: 10 minutes
                                                   Cook time: 20 minutes

I always keep protein bars on me so that if I find myself hungry between meals, I have a healthy snack at the ready. These protein bars also make a great on-the-go breakfast for mornings when you're running behind schedule. The freeze-dried strawberries give this bar a hint of tartness, and the cacao nibs provide a deep chocolatey flavor.

1½ cups sliced almonds
1 cup cashew pieces
½ cup cacao nibs
2 tablespoons unfla-
    vored protein or egg
    white powder
½ teaspoon sea salt
1½ cups Medjool
    dates, pitted
½ cup honey
1 (½-ounce) package
    freeze-dried strawberries
2 tablespoons water

1. Preheat the oven to 325°F and line a 9-by-9-inch baking dish with parchment paper.

2. Place the sliced almonds, cashew pieces, cacao nibs, protein powder, salt, dates, honey, dried strawberries, and water in a food processor and pulse on low speed for 2 minutes. The dates should break down and act as a binder to form a coarse dough. Use a spatula to scrape down the sides of the bowl and pulse for another 30 seconds.

3. Transfer the dough to the baking dish and use the palm of your hand to press it into an even layer. Bake for 20 minutes, then remove it from the oven and allow to cool.

4. Cut the protein bars into 9 equal portions. Store the bars in an airtight container in the refrigerator for up to 1 week or freeze them for up to 6 weeks.

Make It Easier: A quick kitchen hack that works for this recipe and many others: When you're measuring honey, spray the measuring cup with olive oil cooking spray before you put the honey in. The honey will slide right out rather than sticking to the cup.

PER SERVING: *Calories: 343; Total fat: 18g; Sodium: 88mg; Carbohydrates: 46g; Fiber: 4g; Protein: 9g; Iron: 4mg*

Savory Crepes

» Vegetarian

» Serves 2

» Prep time: 10 minutes,
plus 1 hour to rest
Cook time: 10 minutes

Crepes, common in French cuisine, are very thin pancakes that are served with either a sweet or savory filling. Sweet crepes are often eaten as a dessert or snack, whereas savory crepes are frequently served as a meal. Think of this recipe as a blank slate and experiment by using different toppings to create a variety of flavor combinations.

¼ cup plus 1 tablespoon
  tapioca flour
¼ cup almond meal
1 teaspoon coconut flour
2 large eggs
¾ cup unsweetened
  almond milk
⅛ teaspoon sea salt
Olive oil cooking spray, for
  greasing the pan
2 tablespoons sliced
  chives, for garnish
1 tablespoon chopped
  parsley, for garnish

1. Combine the tapioca flour, almond meal, coconut flour, eggs, almond milk, and salt in a blender. Blend on low speed for 2 minutes, until all of the ingredients are fully combined—a smooth batter should form. Rest the batter in the refrigerator for 1 hour, or up to overnight.

2. Heat a small nonstick sauté pan over medium-low heat and coat it with olive oil cooking spray. Pour ¼ cup of batter into the center of the pan and swirl to coat the entire pan with batter. Let cook on the first side for 1 to 2 minutes, until the batter is set and the edges begin to crisp. In a swift motion, flip the crepe and cook for another 1 to 2 minutes. Repeat with the remaining batter.

3. Transfer the crepes to a plate and sprinkle them with chives and parsley. Serve either rolled or folded into triangles.

Ingredient Swaps: Crepes are a versatile base. Try making a sweet version by replacing the herbs with your favorite Paleo-compliant jam. For a dessert treat, add ¼ cup coconut sugar to the batter. Then top the crepes with Paleo-friendly chocolate chips and fresh berries.

PER SERVING: *Calories: 251; Total fat: 12g; Sodium: 195mg; Carbohydrates: 23g; Fiber: 3g; Protein: 12g; Iron: 2mg*

Breakfast Sausage-Stuffed Peppers

» 5-Ingredient, 30 Minutes

» Serves 2

» Prep time: 5 minutes
Cook time: 15 minutes

If you're a fan of breakfast for dinner, this recipe is for you. In this dish, bell peppers act as an edible bowl containing a rich filling of Breakfast Sausage (page 38). Try adding roasted sweet potatoes and baby kale to the egg and sausage mixture for an even more filling meal. To make preparation even easier, cook the sausage in advance and fold it into the scrambled eggs just before the peppers go into the oven.

8 ounces raw Breakfast Sausage (page 38)
2 teaspoons olive oil
3 large eggs
1 tablespoon full-fat coconut milk
½ teaspoon sea salt
¼ teaspoon freshly ground black pepper
1 large red bell pepper or 2 small red bell peppers, halved and deseeded
1 avocado, thinly sliced, for serving

1. Preheat the oven to 400°F.

2. Prepare a half-batch of the Breakfast Sausage (step 1 only).

3. Heat the olive oil in a small sauté pan over medium heat. Add the Breakfast Sausage and cook for 5 minutes, until browned.

4. In a small bowl, combine the eggs and coconut milk and whisk to scramble. Pour the mixture into the sauté pan with the cooked sausage and cook for 1 minute, stirring frequently. Season with salt and pepper.

5. Place the bell pepper halves faceup in an 8-by-8-inch baking dish. Fill the bell pepper halves with the egg and sausage mixture. Bake for 10 minutes, until they start to brown.

6. Remove the peppers from the oven, transfer them to a plate, and top them with avocado slices.

Ingredient Swaps: If you don't eat pork or cannot make the Breakfast Sausage recipe, make this dish with ground beef instead. Try adding diced tomatoes, jalapeño, cumin, paprika, and cilantro for a different flavor profile.

PER SERVING: *Calories: 575; Total fat: 36g; Sodium: 1352mg; Carbohydrates: 28g; Fiber: 11g; Protein: 39g; Iron: 5mg*

Waffles with Espresso Maple Syrup

» 30 Minutes, Vegetarian   » Serves 2   » Prep time: 10 minutes
                                              Cook time: 15 minutes

It is thought that the first waffle iron was invented in Greece to make "hotcakes" between two heated metal plates. National Waffle Day (August 24 in the United States) commemorates the anniversary of the first waffle iron patent—so celebrate with this delicious Paleo-friendly take on traditional waffles. Boost the protein by adding chopped nuts to the batter.

For the waffles

2 tablespoons
   coconut flour
1½ teaspoons ground
   flaxseed (or flax meal)
¼ teaspoon baking soda
1½ teaspoons ground
   cinnamon
⅛ teaspoon sea salt
6 tablespoons
   almond meal
3 large eggs
2 tablespoons honey
½ teaspoon vanilla extract
Olive oil cooking spray, for
   greasing the pan

For the syrup

1 cup maple syrup
2 tablespoons
   instant coffee

1. In a small mixing bowl, combine the coconut flour, flaxseed, baking soda, cinnamon, salt, and almond meal. Stir to combine and set aside

2. In the bowl of a stand mixer fitted with the paddle attachment, combine the eggs, honey, and vanilla. Turn the stand mixer on low speed and slowly add the dry ingredients to the wet. Mix on low for 2 minutes, or until combined.

3. Preheat the waffle iron on medium-high heat. Lightly coat both plates of the iron with olive oil cooking spray. Pour ½ cup of waffle batter into the center of the waffle iron and close the lid. Follow the manufacturer's instructions to cook the waffles, usually 2 to 4 minutes. Use a fork to remove the waffle from the iron and transfer it to a plate. Repeat with remaining batter.

4. **Make the syrup.** In a small bowl, combine the maple syrup and instant coffee. Microwave for 15 seconds, if desired. Drizzle the syrup over the waffles and serve immediately.

5. Refrigerate leftover waffles in an airtight container for up to 4 days or freeze for up to 2 months.

PER SERVING (INCLUDING ¼ CUP SYRUP FOR EACH PORTION): *Calories: 512; Total fat: 17g; Sodium: 361mg; Carbohydrates: 79g; Fiber: 4g; Protein: 15g; Iron: 3mg*

Blueberry-Cardamom Bread Pudding

» Vegetarian, Low-Carb   » Serves 4   » Prep time: 10 minutes
                                        Cook time: 40 minutes

This bread pudding recipe features cardamom, a spice native to Indonesia and made from the seedpods of various plants in the ginger family (its flavor does not resemble ginger). It has a delicate and aromatic flavor that includes notes of citrus, spice, herbs, and mint. Cardamom is thought to offer health benefits, including anti-inflammatory properties, and may aid in digestion, kidney health, and heart-rate regulation. Try switching out the blueberries for any berry of your choice.

Olive oil cooking spray, for greasing the pan

1 loaf day-old Almond Meal Sandwich Bread (page 121), cut into 1-inch cubes

1 cup fresh blueberries

¼ cup pumpkin seeds

5 large eggs

1½ cups full-fat coconut milk

¼ cup maple syrup

2 teaspoons cardamom

½ teaspoon sea salt

1 tablespoon vanilla extract

1. Preheat the oven to 350°F and coat an 8-by-8-inch baking dish with olive oil cooking spray.

2. In a medium bowl, toss the cubed bread, blueberries, and pumpkin seeds to combine, then transfer the mixture to the baking dish.

3. In a separate medium bowl, whisk together the eggs, coconut milk, maple syrup, cardamom, salt, and vanilla. Pour this mixture over the bread mixture. Use a spatula to gently press down on the bread to ensure it soaks up the liquid.

4. Bake the pudding for 30 to 40 minutes, until it is fully set in the center. Serve warm.

Ingredient Swaps: While this recipe is written with fresh blueberries, you can use frozen blueberries (or any other frozen berry) instead.

PER SERVING: *Calories: 1223; Total fat: 98g; Sodium: 1467mg; Carbohydrates: 52g; Fiber: 12g; Protein: 44g; Iron: 11mg*

Crab and Asparagus Omelet

» 5-Ingredient,
30 Minutes, Low-Carb,
Diabetes-Friendly

» Serves 2

» Prep time: 5 minutes
Cook time: 10 minutes

While omelets come in many forms, the two best-known versions are American and French. This recipe makes an American omelet, with a golden crust and uneven craters on the surface. It is folded in half into a half-moon with a rich crabmeat filling in the middle. For the fluffiest possible omelet, mix the eggs in a blender to aerate them.

2 large asparagus spears
2 extra-large eggs
2 tablespoons full-fat coconut milk
1 teaspoon sea salt
¼ teaspoon freshly ground black pepper
2 teaspoons olive oil, divided
½ cup lump crabmeat

1. Set the asparagus on a cutting board, firmly holding it about an inch from the top of the spear. Using a vegetable peeler, shave the asparagus into long, thin strips.

2. Crack the eggs into a blender and add the coconut milk, salt, and pepper. Blend on high for 30 seconds, until light and fluffy.

3. Heat 1 teaspoon of olive oil in a small nonstock sauté pan over medium-low heat until the oil is shimmering. Add the asparagus peelings to the pan and sauté for 1 minute. Remove the asparagus from the pan and set aside.

4. Add the remaining 1 teaspoon of olive oil to the pan, raise the heat to medium, and pour in the egg mixture. Using a heat-resistant rubber spatula, gently push the edge of the eggs toward the center of the pan, slightly tilting the pan so the uncooked egg flows back to the edges. Continue around the edges of the pan until no liquid remains and the eggs are just set.

5. Remove the pan from heat and place the asparagus strips and crabmeat on one half of the omelet. Using the spatula, gently fold the omelet in half. Cut in half and serve immediately.

PER SERVING: *Calories: 181; Total fat: 13g; Sodium: 853mg; Carbohydrates: 2g; Fiber: 0g; Protein: 14g; Iron: 2mg*

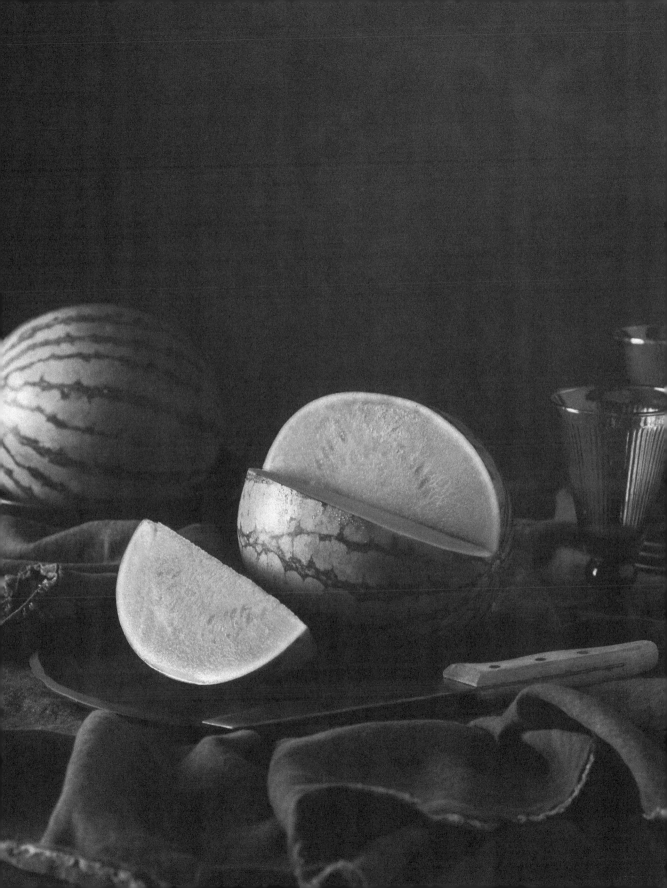

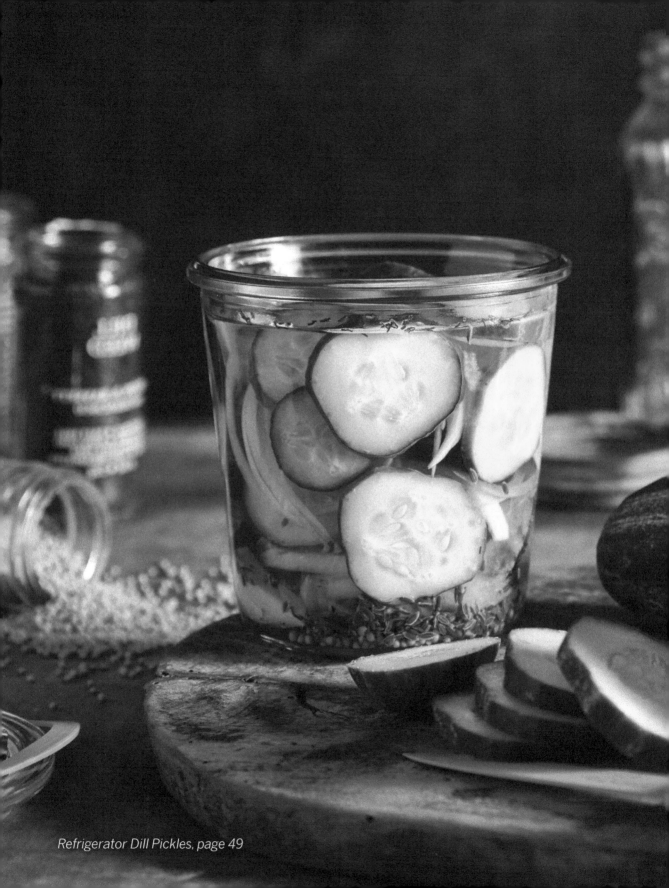

Refrigerator Dill Pickles, page 49

CHAPTER FOUR

Snacks and Sides

On the Paleo diet, preparation is the key to success. Many of us lead busy lives, and unfortunately, the snack foods at our disposal—whether French fries from the drive-through, chips from the gas station, or candy from the vending machine—are often unhealthy. For this reason, keeping healthy snacks on hand and readily available is key to reducing our dependence on unhealthy store-bought snacks. Chocolate-Banana Trail Mix (page 56) is a perfect alternative to a candy bar—it offers a sweet chocolate component without high sugar and preservatives. Everything Seed Crackers (page 55) and Bacon-Jalapeño Guacamole (page 52) make great afternoon snacks. Dive into this chapter to find a plethora of healthy alternatives for side dishes and snacking.

Refrigerator Dill Pickles

» Low-Carb, One-Pot, Vegetarian

» Makes 4 cups

» Prep time: 20 minutes, plus 24 hours to chill

There are a few different types of cucumbers, and the most common are slicing cucumbers and pickling cucumbers. Slicing cucumbers are usually large with a thin skin, while pickling cucumbers are smaller with a thick skin. For this recipe, be sure to use pickling cucumbers, such as Kirby or Persian cucumbers, whose thick skins will produce crispy, crunchy pickles. For extra-crunchy pickles, try adding grape leaves, which release tannins that can prevent your pickles from softening.

2 pounds seedless thick-skinned cucumbers, sliced into ¼-inch rounds

1 small sweet onion, julienned

2½ cups water

2 garlic cloves, finely chopped

1 tablespoon sea salt

1 tablespoon mustard seeds

2 teaspoons dried dill

2 teaspoons coconut sugar

1 teaspoon dill seeds (optional)

6 dried bay leaves (optional)

2½ cups apple cider vinegar

1. In a large glass jar with a lid, combine the cucumbers, onion, water, garlic, salt, mustard seeds, dill, coconut sugar, dill seeds (if using), and bay leaves (if using).

2. In a small saucepan over medium heat, bring the apple cider vinegar to a boil. Once boiling, pour the vinegar into the jar over the cucumber mixture.

3. Allow the cucumber and vinegar mixture to cool for 1 hour at room temperature, then seal the container. Refrigerate the pickles for at least 24 hours before serving.

Scale It Up: These pickles can be stored in the refrigerator for up to 2 months, making them a great snack or side to keep on hand. You can double or even triple the recipe to make a larger batch.

PER SERVING: *Calories: 40; Total fat: 0g; Sodium: 297mg; Carbohydrates: 9g; Fiber: 1g; Protein: 1g; Iron: 1mg*

Creamy Kale Slaw

» One-Pot, 30 Minutes, Vegetarian, Diabetes-Friendly

» Makes 4 cups

» Prep time: 15 minutes

Kale is full of antioxidants, essential nutrients, and vitamins C, K, A, and B, as well as manganese. There are several types of kale—curly kale is a common variety, as is dinosaur kale, which has long, bumpy leaves. Our favorite is Red Russian kale, with hardy, tender leaves and purplish-red stalks. Any of these varieties will work for this versatile side. To make prep easier, make the dressing ahead and keep it refrigerated until you're ready to put everything together.

½ cup Paleo Mayo (page 156)

2 tablespoons coconut sugar

1½ tablespoons freshly squeezed lemon juice

1 tablespoon apple cider vinegar

1 tablespoon celery seed

½ teaspoon sea salt

½ teaspoon freshly ground black pepper

2 cups shredded cabbage

2 cups chopped kale

1 tablespoon sunflower seeds

1. Prepare the mayo.

2. **Make the dressing.** In a small bowl, whisk together the mayo, coconut sugar, lemon juice, vinegar, celery seed, salt, and pepper until smooth and creamy.

3. In a medium bowl, combine the shredded cabbage, chopped kale, and sunflower seeds.

4. Pour the dressing over the kale and cabbage and mix thoroughly to coat. Serve cold and refrigerate leftovers for up to 4 days in an airtight container.

Scale It Up: Double or triple this recipe for a crowd or to enjoy all week—it makes a great side for a picnic lunch, whether you follow the Paleo diet or not.

PER SERVING: *Calories: 142; Total fat: 13g; Sodium: 137mg; Carbohydrates: 7g; Fiber: 1g; Protein: 1g; Iron: 1mg*

Baked Buffalo Cauliflower

» 5-Ingredient,
Vegetarian, Low-Carb,
Diabetes-Friendly

» Serves 2

» Prep time: 5 minutes
Cook time: 25 minutes

Buffalo cauliflower is a healthy spin on buffalo wings—a nutritious base with the same heat. There are several commercial hot sauces available that are Paleo-friendly. Our favorite brands are Frank's RedHot, Tabasco Habanero Pepper Sauce, and Trader Joe's Habanero Hot Sauce. This dish pairs perfectly with Guilt-Free Ranch Dressing (page 160) or the dressing from Classic Wedge Salad with "Bleu Cheese" Dressing (page 71). Serve with carrots and celery to round out the dish.

1 small head cauliflower,
cut into bite-size florets
1 tablespoon olive oil
½ cup Paleo-compliant hot
sauce of your choice

1. Preheat the oven to 400°F and line a baking sheet with parchment paper.

2. In a medium bowl, toss the cauliflower florets with the olive oil. Transfer the cauliflower to the baking sheet and roast for 15 minutes.

3. While the cauliflower roasts, heat the hot sauce in a small sauté pan over low heat. Simmer for 10 minutes, until the sauce thickens and reduces in volume.

4. Remove the baking sheet from the oven and drizzle the hot sauce over the cauliflower, tossing to coat. Return the cauliflower to the oven and roast for 10 minutes, until the sauce begins to char and the cauliflower is tender. Serve hot.

Ingredient Swaps: You can customize the spice level in this dish by increasing or decreasing amount of hot sauce used, or try switching the hot sauce out for a milder or spicier Paleo-compliant sauce.

PER SERVING: *Calories: 100; Total fat: 8g; Sodium: 404mg; Carbohydrates: 7g; Fiber: 3g; Protein: 3g; Iron: 1mg*

Bacon-Jalapeño Guacamole

» 30 Minutes, Low-Carb, Diabetes-Friendly

» Serves 2

» Prep time: 15 minutes

Avocados are packed with oleic fatty acid, a healthy fat that has been shown to reduce inflammation. Like many fruits, they are also full of vitamins and minerals and actually contain more potassium than bananas. Avocados provide a rich and filling base for this snack, great for refueling after a workout. They can be bland on their own, but the added citrus, acidity, and fresh herbs in this recipe make their flavor pop.

6 slices bacon

3 large avocados, peeled and seeded

Zest and juice of 1 lime

1 teaspoon sea salt

¼ teaspoon freshly ground black pepper

1 medium jalapeño, seeded and diced

½ yellow onion, diced

2 Roma tomatoes, diced

3 tablespoons chopped fresh cilantro

1. Cook the bacon in a medium sauté pan over medium heat for about 3 minutes on each side. Set the cooked bacon on a plate with a paper towel to cool. The paper towel will absorb excess grease.

2. In a medium bowl, combine the avocados, lime zest and juice, salt, and pepper. Use a fork to mash the avocados. Stir in the jalapeño, onion, tomatoes, and cilantro.

3. Once the bacon is cool, dice it and fold it into the avocado mixture. Serve immediately or refrigerate in an airtight container for up to 1 day.

Scale It Up: Double this guacamole recipe to serve a crowd or to use in several other dishes. Try it with Tortilla Chips (page 125), Tilapia Fish Tacos (page 113), or as a snack served with sliced bell peppers.

PER SERVING: *Calories: 750; Total fat: 58g; Sodium: 1032mg; Carbohydrates: 46g; Fiber: 28g; Protein: 23g; Iron: 2mg*

Baba Ghanoush

» Vegetarian, Low-Carb, Diabetes-Friendly

» Serves 2

» Prep time: 10 minutes
Cook time: 30 minutes

Baba ghanoush is an appetizer with origins in the Levant, a historical region in the modern-day Middle East. It is usually made with eggplant and olive oil, but ingredients vary by region. Our Paleo-friendly take on the dish adds a bit of smoke and has an almost hummus-like consistency.

1 large eggplant, cut in half lengthways

4 tablespoons olive oil, divided

2 teaspoons sea salt

½ teaspoon freshly ground black pepper

1 tablespoon minced garlic

¼ cup tahini

½ teaspoon ground cumin

Zest and juice of 1 large lemon

2 tablespoons chopped fresh cilantro, for garnish

Pinch paprika, sumac, or za'atar, for garnish

1. Preheat the oven to 400°F and line a baking sheet with aluminum foil.

2. Use a knife to score the flesh of the eggplant in a crisscross pattern, cutting grooves about 1 inch deep. Coat the scored sides of the eggplant with 2 tablespoons olive oil and season them with salt and pepper.

3. Place the eggplant on the baking sheet, cut-side down, and roast for 30 minutes, or until soft. Remove from the oven and allow to cool. Once the eggplant is cool enough to handle, peel its skin off using your fingers or a knife (it should come off easily).

4. In the bowl of a food processor, combine the roasted eggplant, garlic, tahini, cumin, the remaining 2 tablespoons olive oil, and lemon zest and juice. Process on high until a thick, smooth paste forms. Transfer to a serving dish and garnish with cilantro and paprika, sumac, or za'atar. Serve at room temperature or chilled. Refrigerate leftovers for up to 4 days.

Scale It Up: Double or triple this recipe to serve a crowd. I recommend serving it with Tortilla Chips (page 125), Everything Seed Crackers (page 55), or sliced bell peppers for a perfect midday snack.

PER SERVING: *Calories: 500; Total fat: 44g; Sodium: 1206mg; Carbohydrates: 26g; Fiber: 11g; Protein: 8g; Iron: 4mg*

Cauliflower "Rice"

» One-Pot, 30 Minutes, Vegetarian, Low-Carb, Diabetes-Friendly

» Serves 2

» Prep time: 10 minutes
Cook time: 10 minutes

In recent years, riced cauliflower has emerged as a welcome substitute for white rice, which is starchy and high in carbohydrates. The trick to good cauliflower rice is in the preparation. Use a food processor to grate the cauliflower to ensure it cooks evenly. Be careful not to overcook it, as it will lose texture and become mushy. Many stores sell packaged pre-riced cauliflower, which can save you valuable prep time and get dinner on the table faster.

1 head cauliflower (or 1 [16-ounce] package riced cauliflower)

1 tablespoon olive oil

1 teaspoon sea salt

½ teaspoon freshly ground black pepper

1 tablespoon minced garlic

Juice of 1 lime

2 tablespoons chopped scallions

2 tablespoons fresh chopped cilantro

½ teaspoon ground coriander

1. Trim the cauliflower to remove as much stem as possible. Cut the trimmed cauliflower into small sections and transfer to a food processor. Process on low speed for 2 minutes, stopping periodically to ensure larger chunks are being processed. Look for pieces the size of a grain of rice.

2. Heat the olive oil in a large sauté pan over medium heat. Add the cauliflower, salt, and pepper and cook for 6 to 8 minutes, stirring occasionally, until the cauliflower softens and begins to brown. Add the minced garlic and cook for 2 minutes.

3. Remove the cauliflower from the heat and transfer it to a medium bowl. Add the lime juice, scallions, cilantro, and ground coriander and stir to coat. Serve immediately or refrigerate for up to 3 days in an airtight container.

Scale It Up: This dish can be served with so many different entrées, so make a double batch for easier prep later in the week. Serve with Seared Mahi-Mahi with Coconut-Caper Sauce (page 103), Ginger-Beef Stir-Fry (page 105), or Tandoori-Style Chicken (page 104).

PER SERVING: *Calories: 131; Total fat: 8g; Sodium: 652mg; Carbohydrates: 15g; Fiber: 5g; Protein: 5g; Iron: 1mg*

Everything Seed Crackers

» Low-Carb,
Diabetes-Friendly

» Serves 4

» Prep time: 10 minutes
Cook time: 30 minutes

Flaxseed is one of the oldest crops known to man: Even Hippocrates used flaxseed to aid digestion. Flaxseed is high in fiber, protein, and omega-3 fatty acids and has also gained popularity recently as a quick and easy substitute for eggs as a binder in baking.

1 cup flaxseed meal

1 tablespoon dried minced garlic

1 tablespoon dried minced onion

2 tablespoons black sesame seeds

2 tablespoons white sesame seeds

2 tablespoons poppy seeds

½ teaspoon sea salt

¾ cup water

1 tablespoon freshly squeezed lemon juice

1. Preheat the oven to 350°F.

2. In a medium bowl, combine the flaxseed meal, garlic, onion, black and white sesame seeds, poppy seeds, and salt. Stir to combine.

3. Slowly add the water and lemon juice to the flaxseed mixture, using a spatula to stir continuously. As the mixture starts to form a dough, it may be easier to mix with your hands. Once fully mixed, you should be able to form a cohesive ball of dough.

4. Place the dough ball between two sheets of parchment paper and press it to flatten slightly. Using a rolling pin, roll the dough out as thin as possible (about ⅛ inch or thinner).

5. Remove the top sheet of parchment paper and use a knife or pizza cutter to slice the dough into 2-inch triangles or squares.

6. Transfer the parchment paper with the cracker dough to a baking sheet. Bake for 25 minutes, or until the crackers are dry in the center. Remove from the oven, let cool, and then break apart at the cut lines. Store in an airtight container for up to 4 days.

PER SERVING: *Calories: 228; Total fat: 19g; Sodium: 159mg; Carbohydrates: 11g; Fiber: 10g; Protein: 8g; Iron: 3mg*

Chocolate-Banana Trail Mix

» 30 Minutes, Vegetarian » Serves 2 » Prep time: 5 minutes
Cook time: 25 minutes

Trail mix, sometimes called "gorp," is a staple for us. It's perfect for snacking on a hike, at work, or to keep in the car as an emergency snack. You can make trail mix with any nuts, seeds, and dried fruit you have on hand. We recommend purchasing dried fruits and nuts from Nuts.com—always check that dried fruits are unsweetened and free of preservatives. Switch this recipe up with different ingredients to make brand-new versions every time.

1 cup unsweetened
  banana chips
½ cup cacao nibs
½ cup pumpkin seeds
½ cup sunflower seeds
½ cup apricot kernels
½ teaspoon sea salt
½ teaspoon cinnamon
1 teaspoon vanilla extract
2 tablespoons honey
2 tablespoons
  almond butter

1. Preheat the oven to 300°F and line a baking sheet with parchment paper.

2. In a medium bowl, combine the banana chips, cacao nibs, pumpkin seeds, sunflower seeds, apricot kernels, salt, and cinnamon.

3. In a small bowl, combine the vanilla, honey, and almond butter. Pour this mixture over the seed mixture and toss to coat evenly.

4. Spread the trail mix in a thin layer on the baking sheet. Bake for 20 minutes, stirring halfway through to ensure even browning. Serve immediately or store in an airtight container for up to 1 month.

Ingredient Swaps: An apricot kernel is the seed of an apricot and has a slightly nutty, slightly sweet flavor. If you can't find apricot kernels, you can substitute an equal amount of raw almonds.

PER SERVING: *Calories: 1072; Total fat: 76g; Sodium: 314mg; Carbohydrates: 92g; Fiber: 16g; Protein: 34g; Iron: 18mg*

Asparagus Amandine

» 30 Minutes,
  5-Ingredient,
  Vegetarian, Low-Carb,
  Diabetes-Friendly

» Serves 2

» Prep time: 5 minutes
  Cook time: 15 minutes

Asparagus comes in green, white, and purple hues, but all colors have similar flavor profiles. A single spear of asparagus contains just 4 calories and is rich in fiber, folate, potassium, and vitamins E, A, C and K. Asparagus is in season from April through late June, so this sautéed dish with toasted almonds is a great dish for springtime.

1 cup plus 1 tablespoon
  water, divided
1 tablespoon plus
  1 teaspoon sea
  salt, divided
1 bunch asparagus
  (roughly 1 pound)
2 tablespoons olive oil
1½ teaspoons
  garlic, minced
1 tablespoon shallot,
  minced
2 teaspoons freshly ground
  black pepper
¼ cup toasted almonds

1. Blanch the asparagus. In a saucepan or pot, bring 1 cup water to a boil and add 1 tablespoon salt. Add the asparagus to the saucepan and allow it to boil for 1 minute. You should see the asparagus brighten and intensify in color. Quickly remove the asparagus from the water to avoid overcooking and set it aside.

2. Heat the olive oil in a large sauté pan over low heat. Add the garlic and shallot and cook for 2 minutes, stirring occasionally, until just golden and fragrant.

3. Add the blanched asparagus to the pan and cook for 2 minutes, stirring frequently. Add the remaining 1 teaspoon salt, black pepper, almonds, and the remaining 1 tablespoon water. Toss everything together to coat. Remove from heat and serve immediately.

Ingredient Swaps: Most legumes are not permitted on the Paleo diet, but green beans are an exception. Green beans do not have the inflammatory properties of most other legumes, so they are allowed. For a different flavor profile, try this recipe using green beans in place of asparagus.

PER SERVING: *Calories: 275; Total fat: 23g; Sodium: 587mg; Carbohydrates: 14g; Fiber: 7g; Protein: 9g; Iron: 6mg*

Truffle Parsnip Fries

» One-Pot, 30 Minutes, 5-Ingredient, Vegetarian, Low-Carb

» Serves 2

» Prep time: 5 minutes
Cook time: 25 minutes

When we switched to the Paleo diet, one the foods we missed most was French fries. Luckily, we found a Paleo-friendly replacement to satisfy our cravings. These delicious fries are made with parsnips instead of potatoes and are oven-roasted rather than deep-fried. The secret to this recipe is quickly broiling the parsnip fries after roasting to achieve a crispy-on-the-outside, soft-on-the-inside texture. Sweet potatoes roasted the same way make another substitute for French fries.

3 to 5 medium parsnips, peeled and cut into thin French fry–like strips

2 tablespoons olive oil

2 teaspoons truffle oil

2 teaspoons sea salt

1 teaspoon freshly ground black pepper

½ teaspoon paprika, for garnish

1. Preheat the oven to 425°F and line a large baking sheet with parchment paper.

2. In a medium bowl, toss the parsnips with the olive oil and truffle oil to coat evenly.

3. Spread the parsnips in a single layer on the baking sheet and sprinkle them with salt and pepper. Roast for 10 minutes, then flip them and continue roasting for an additional 10 to 15 minutes, or until they are tender. Switch the oven to broil and broil on high for 2 minutes, or until crisp.

4. Remove the baking sheet from the oven and sprinkle the fries with paprika. Serve immediately.

Ingredient Swaps: Truffles, a type of fungus, grow in the shadows of oak trees and are considered a delicacy in many cuisines. They have a very distinctive odor and flavor, and a little bit goes a long way. If you don't have truffle oil on hand, you can easily omit it and still come out with a delicious dish.

PER SERVING: *Calories: 409; Total fat: 19g; Sodium: 1197mg; Carbohydrates: 60g; Fiber: 17g; Protein: 4g; Iron: 2mg*

Game-Day Chicken Wings

» Low-Carb,
  Diabetes-Friendly

» Serves 4

» Prep time: 5 minutes
  Cook time: 25 minutes

The game is on, perhaps some friends are gathered around, and you're ready to snack. This situation seems like an easy way to stray from the Paleo diet, but we have you covered with this Paleo-friendly game-day dish. Serve these wings with Tortilla Chips (page 125), Bacon-Jalapeño Guacamole (page 52), and sliced vegetables with Baba Ghanoush (page 53) to put together an ultimate game day spread.

2 teaspoons sea salt
2 tablespoons freshly
  ground black pepper
1 teaspoon cayenne pepper
½ teaspoon cumin
1 tablespoon chili powder
2 tablespoons tapioca
  starch
3 or 4 pounds
  chicken wings
¼ cup Paleo-compliant hot
  sauce (such as Tabasco
  or Frank's RedHot)

1. Preheat the oven to 425°F and line a baking sheet with aluminum foil.

2. Make the seasoning blend. In a small mixing bowl, combine the salt, black pepper, cayenne pepper, cumin, chili powder, and tapioca starch. Whisk together with a fork to incorporate.

3. Place the chicken wings in a large mixing bowl and sprinkle them with the seasoning blend. Rub the seasoning into the wings, making sure they are liberally covered.

4. Transfer the seasoned wings to the baking sheet and spread in a single layer. Bake for 15 minutes, then flip them and continue baking for an additional 10 minutes.

5. Remove the wings from the oven and place them in a separate bowl. Pour in the hot sauce and any juices left over from cooking and toss to coat. Serve immediately. To reheat or crisp up the chicken wings, place under the broiler for 2 minutes or bake at 400°F for 10 minutes.

Scale It Up: Double this recipe to feed a crowd or to have leftovers for lunch the next day.

PER SERVING: *Calories: 876; Total fat: 59g; Sodium: 657mg; Carbohydrates: 1g; Fiber: 0g; Protein: 81g; Iron: 4mg*

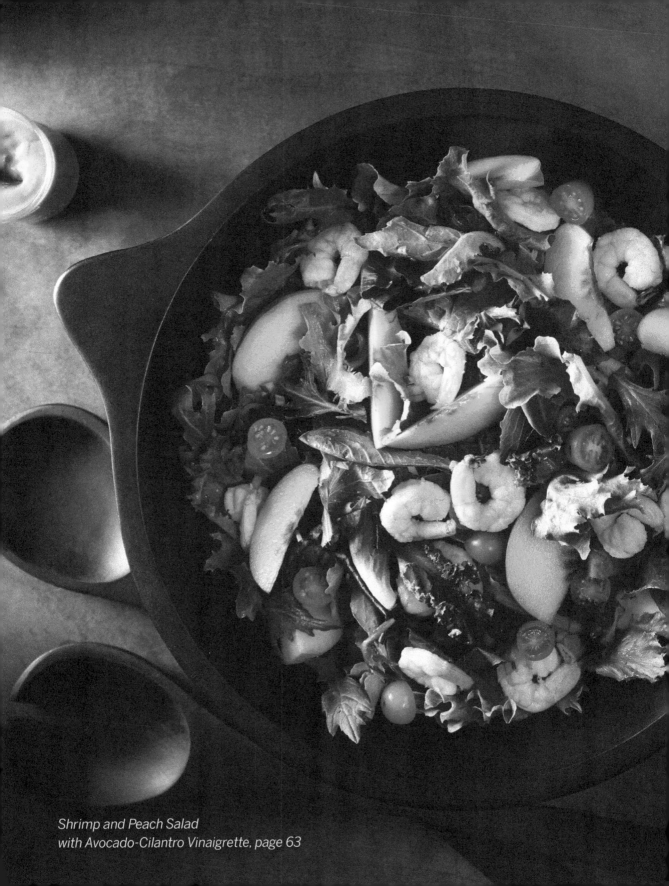

Shrimp and Peach Salad
with Avocado-Cilantro Vinaigrette, page 63

CHAPTER FIVE

Salads

—◇—

Salads don't have to be boring—when prepared well, they can be the most flavorful and nutrient-diverse dishes out there. Salads carry the unfortunate and inaccurate reputation of being "rabbit food." In this chapter, we challenge those assumptions by offering delicious and hearty salads that will fill you up and delight your taste buds. A nutritious, filling salad needs to be more than just leafy greens—it should include a full serving of protein and healthy fats (try adding sliced roasted chicken and avocado to your next salad to boost its nutrient value). Salads are also often considered to be a spring or summer dish only, but you can enjoy them year-round. This chapter includes several salads that feature warm autumnal or wintery vegetables, including the Beet and Carrot Salad with Black Pepper Vinaigrette (page 67) and the Winter Squash Salad with Spiced Maple Vinaigrette (page 74). Many of our salad recipes include recipes for dressings or vinaigrettes, many of which keep in the refrigerator for up to a month—make a full batch and enjoy it on salads for weeks!

Shrimp and Peach Salad with Avocado-Cilantro Vinaigrette

» 30 Minutes, Low-Carb   » Serves 2   » Prep time: 10 minutes
Cook time: 5 minutes

In this fragrant salad, the shrimp are poached, which keeps them very tender and juicy. Putting the shrimp in the refrigerator immediately after cooking halts the cooking process, keeping them from becoming tough. Peaches are in season from late June through August, so make this salad in summertime.

For the shrimp

3 quarts water
3 tablespoons Old Bay seasoning
3 tablespoons sea salt
Juice of 1 lemon
3 garlic cloves, minced
½ yellow onion, chopped
1 bay leaf
1 thyme sprig
1 pound shrimp, peeled and deveined, tails removed

For the salad

2 tablespoons Avocado-Cilantro Vinaigrette (page 155)
3 cups mixed leafy greens
1 small shallot, diced
1 peach, cut into segments
½ cup cherry tomatoes, halved

1. Prepare the vinaigrette.

2. In a medium pot, bring the water to a boil over high heat. Add the Old Bay, salt, lemon juice, garlic, onion, bay leaf, and thyme over high heat.

3. Once the water reaches a rolling boil, add the shrimp to the pot and reduce the heat to a simmer. Poach the shrimp for 60 to 90 seconds—they should become opaque. Quickly drain and discard the liquid and transfer the shrimp to a bowl. Place in the refrigerator.

4. While the shrimp cool, make the salad. Combine the mixed greens in a bowl with the shallots, peach, and cherry tomatoes. Add the vinaigrette and toss to coat.

5. Divide the dressed greens between two plates and top with cooled shrimp. Serve immediately or refrigerate the shrimp, salad, and dressing separately in airtight containers for up to 3 days.

Make It Easier: We recommend preparing the shrimp for this recipe up to 3 days ahead to make for a quick and easy lunch or dinner.

PER SERVING: *Calories: 284; Total fat: 2g; Sodium: 862mg; Carbohydrates: 21g; Fiber: 4g; Protein: 48g; Iron: 3mg*

Pork Belly and Watermelon Salad with Ginger-Peach Dressing

» 30 Minutes

» Serves 2

» Prep time: 10 minutes
Cook time: 20 minutes

Pork belly is most often used in the United States to make bacon, but we use it in its uncured form in this recipe. Pork belly is usually prepared by braising over low-and-slow heat before searing it until crispy in a skillet. In this rich but refreshing salad, we use a quick-roast method instead of braising to cut down on cooking time while maintaining a tender, flavorful result.

For the dressing

2 peaches, peeled, halved, and pitted
¼ cup olive oil
½ cup apple cider vinegar
2 tablespoons honey
2 teaspoons freshly grated ginger
1 teaspoon sea salt
¼ teaspoon curry powder (optional)

For the salad

1 pound pork belly, cut into 1-inch strips
3 cups watermelon, cubed
1 large shallot, sliced into rings
2 cups arugula
2 mint sprigs, leaves only
2 small radishes, thinly sliced, for garnish (optional)
1 small jalapeño, thinly sliced, for garnish (optional)
1 tablespoon sesame seeds, for garnish (optional)

1. Preheat the oven to 450°F and line a baking sheet with aluminum foil.

2. Lay the pork belly pieces on the baking sheet in a single layer. Roast for 20 minutes, or until brown, crispy and fully rendered. Remove from the oven and set aside to cool.

3. **While the pork belly roasts, make the dressing.** In a blender, combine the peaches, olive oil, vinegar, honey, ginger, salt, and curry powder (if using). Blend on high speed until smooth.

4. **Make the salad.** In a large mixing bowl, combine the watermelon, shallot, arugula, mint, and cooled pork belly. Toss the salad to combine, then transfer it to two plates for serving. Liberally spoon the dressing over the salad and garnish with radishes, jalapeño, and sesame seeds (if using).

Ingredient Swaps: If you cannot find pork belly at your grocer, you can use thick-cut bacon in its place—just make sure it is uncured and contains no added sugar or nitrates.

PER SERVING: *Calories: 1649; Total fat: 148g; Sodium: 669mg; Carbohydrates: 59g; Fiber: 4g; Protein: 25g; Iron: 3mg*

Easy Cucumber and Tomato Salad

» One-Pot, 30 Minutes, 5-Ingredient, Vegetarian, Low-Carb, Diabetes-Friendly

» Serves 2

» Prep time: 15 minutes

While we use pickling cucumbers in the Refrigerator Dill Pickles (page 49), here we use an English cucumber with a thin skin perfect for snacking on raw. Cucumbers have a high water content, which makes this a great recipe to keep you hydrated on a hot summer day. If you're making this recipe ahead, consider storing the salad separately from the vinaigrette—dress the salad just before serving.

3 tablespoons Basic Vinaigrette (page 153)

1 English cucumber, cut into 1-inch chunks

1 cup cherry tomatoes, halved

1 small shallot, sliced

1 tablespoon fresh dill, chopped

½ teaspoon sea salt

¼ teaspoon freshly ground black pepper

1. Prepare the vinaigrette.

2. Combine the cucumber, tomatoes, shallot, dill, salt, and pepper in a small bowl. Add the vinaigrette and toss to coat. Serve immediately at room temperature or chilled. Refrigerate leftovers for up to 2 days in an airtight container.

Scale It Up: You can double or even triple this recipe to serve a group or to enjoy all weekend. This makes a great summer salad for a picnic or barbecue.

PER SERVING: *Calories: 185; Total fat: 16g; Sodium: 300mg; Carbohydrates: 11g; Fiber: 3g; Protein: 2g; Iron: 1mg*

Beet and Carrot Salad with Black Pepper Vinaigrette

» 30 Minutes,
Vegetarian, Low-Carb,
Diabetes-Friendly

» Serves 2

» Prep time: 15 minutes

Beets are considered a "superfood" and are high in nutrition and low in calories. Consuming beets has been shown to lower blood pressure and to support athletic performance by improving blood nitrate levels (levels peak 2 to 3 hours after eating). Beets can be enjoyed numerous ways, including raw, juiced, roasted, steamed, or boiled. In this refreshing salad, raw beet "zoodles" are the star of the show.

For the dressing

1/3 cup freshly squeezed
   lemon juice
2/3 cup olive oil
1 tablespoon maple syrup
1 teaspoon freshly ground
   black pepper
1 teaspoon Dijon mustard
1/2 teaspoon sea salt

For the salad

2 mint sprigs, leaves only
1/3 pound raw red
   beet zoodles
3/4 cup carrots, shredded
1 shallot, thinly sliced
   into rings
4 cups mixed baby greens

1. **Make the dressing.** Combine the lemon juice, olive oil, maple syrup, black pepper, mustard, and salt in a jar with an airtight lid and seal. Shake vigorously for 15 to 20 seconds, until combined. The vinaigrette will separate after a few minutes, but you can shake it to recombine once ready to use.

2. **Make the salad.** Tear the mint leaves in half. Add the beet zoodles, carrots, shallot, and mixed baby greens to a large mixing bowl and toss to combine. Shake the vinaigrette again and pour 3 tablespoons over the salad. Toss again to coat and serve immediately. Keep any remaining salad dressing in the jar and refrigerate for up to 2 weeks.

Make It Easier: Spiralized vegetable noodles are growing in popularity and are increasingly available at supermarkets. Check your grocery store's produce section for spiralized beets to make this recipe quick and easy.

PER SERVING: *Calories: 260; Total fat: 21g; Sodium: 200mg; Carbohydrates: 18g; Fiber: 5g; Protein: 3g; Iron: 2mg*

Baby Kale Salad with Chipotle Caesar Dressing

» 30 Minutes, Low-Carb, Diabetes-Friendly

» Serves 2

» Prep time: 15 minutes

Our unique take on Caesar salad has spicy chipotle peppers in adobo sauce and toasted almonds, which offer subtle sweetness. We also use baby kale instead of romaine, since it is nutrient-dense and packed with vitamins.

For the dressing

8 large egg yolks
2 teaspoons sea salt
1 cup olive oil
1 tablespoon chipotle peppers
2 tablespoons full-fat coconut milk
1 tablespoon anchovies
1 tablespoon freshly squeezed lemon juice
2 teaspoons minced garlic
1½ teaspoons granulated onion
1½ teaspoons Dijon mustard
½ teaspoon black pepper

For the salad

½ cup Garlic-Herb Bread Crumbs (page 127)
4 cups baby kale
¼ cup toasted almonds

1. Make the bread crumbs, if necessary.

2. **Make the dressing.** Place the egg yolks and salt in the bowl of a food processor. Turn the processor on and drizzle in the olive oil in a slow, steady stream.

3. Stop the processor and add the chipotle peppers, coconut milk, anchovies, lemon juice, garlic, onion, mustard, and black pepper. Process for 2 minutes, or until smooth.

4. **Make the salad.** Combine the baby kale, almonds, and bread crumbs in a medium bowl. Add 3 tablespoons dressing and toss to coat. Serve immediately.

5. Refrigerate any remaining dressing in an airtight container for up to 1 week.

PER SERVING: *Calories: 489; Total fat: 41g; Sodium: 518mg; Carbohydrates: 17g; Fiber: 6g; Protein: 14g; Iron: 3mg*

Summer Citrus Salad with Sweet Tea Vinaigrette

» 30 Minutes, Vegetarian   » Serves 2   » Prep time: 20 minutes

We live in the South, where sweet tea rules the beverage world. Unfortunately, most sweet tea has a ton of sugar and a high calorie count. For this recipe, we were inspired by sweet tea to make a healthy tea-infused vinaigrette. For the supremes, you want to peel away the skin and white pith of the orange first, and then run the knife down the edge of the membrane to release each segment.

For the dressing

2 cups brewed
   unsweetened tea
2 tablespoons
   Dijon mustard
2 tablespoons honey
¼ cup apple cider vinegar
1 teaspoon sea salt
1 teaspoon white pepper
¾ cup olive oil

For the salad

4 cups mixed greens
¼ cup thinly sliced
   fennel bulb
1 orange, cut into
   supremes
½ grapefruit, cut into
   supremes

1. **Make the dressing.** Combine the tea, mustard, honey, apple cider vinegar, salt, and white pepper in a blender. Blend on medium speed and slowly drizzle in the olive oil in an even stream. Continue blending to emulsify—the vinaigrette should look creamy.

2. **Make the salad.** In a medium bowl, toss the mixed greens, shaved fennel, orange supremes, and grapefruit supremes. Add 2 tablespoons vinaigrette and toss to coat. Serve immediately and refrigerate the extra vinaigrette in an airtight jar for up to 1 month.

Make It Easier: Some oranges are easier to peel and segment than others. If you don't have time to cut the oranges into supremes, use a Sumo Citrus (sometimes called a dekopon) instead—its segments are easy to peel apart and toss into the salad quickly. If you can't find a Sumo Citrus, try using any seedless clementine.

PER SERVING: *Calories: 172; Total fat: 10g; Sodium: 107mg; Carbohydrates: 20g; Fiber: 4g; Protein: 3g; Iron: 2mg*

Roasted Fig Salad with Maple-Tahini Dressing

» 30 Minutes, Vegetarian   » Serves 2   » Prep time: 15 minutes
Cook time: 15 minutes

Fresh figs, which form the base of this dish, have a soft texture and a sweet, honey-like flavor. They are in season for a short time in early summer and again from the end of summer through the beginning of fall. We recommend making this salad when you can get fresh, in-season figs. The figs in this salad are complemented by maple syrup and tahini, an earthy, nutty spread made from hulled sesame seeds.

For the roasted figs

10 fresh figs, halved
1 teaspoon sea salt

For the dressing

¼ cup tahini
1 tablespoon Dijon mustard
1 tablespoon maple syrup
1 tablespoon
    sherry vinegar
1 tablespoon warm water
1 teaspoon sea salt

For the salad

½ small red onion,
    thinly sliced
4 cups mixed greens
¼ cup toasted pecans,
    for garnish

1. Preheat the oven to 425°F and line a baking sheet with parchment paper.

2. Place the figs on the baking sheet, cut-side up, and sprinkle them with 1 teaspoon sea salt. Roast them for 10 to 12 minutes, until they begin to blister and bubble. Remove them from the oven and set aside.

3. While the figs roast, make the dressing. In a small bowl, whisk together the tahini, mustard, maple syrup, sherry vinegar, water, and salt.

4. **Make the salad.** In a large bowl, toss the red onion and mixed greens with 3 tablespoons dressing. Transfer the salad to two plates, top them with roasted figs, and then garnish with pecans. Serve immediately. Refrigerate the extra salad dressing in an airtight jar for up to 2 weeks.

Ingredient Swaps: If fresh figs are not in season, you can use dried figs instead. Chop the same amount of dried figs into bite-size pieces and toss them with the other ingredients before serving.

PER SERVING: *Calories: 370; Total fat: 17g; Sodium: 735mg; Carbohydrates: 59g; Fiber: 12g; Protein: 7g; Iron: 4mg*

Classic Wedge Salad with "Bleu Cheese" Dressing

» 30 Minutes, Low-Carb, Diabetes-Friendly

» Serves 4

» Prep time: 15 minutes

Wedge salads first became popular in the late 1950s, and they are what they sound like: a "wedge" cut out of a head of iceberg lettuce. While bleu cheese itself is not Paleo-compliant, we created a dressing to mimic its flavor using vinegar, tarragon, and nutritional yeast, an often-overlooked but very useful ingredient that offers a deep, almost cheesy flavor. We use it as a Paleo-friendly stand-in in several recipes elsewhere in this book.

For the dressing

1 cup Paleo Mayo (page 156)

2 tablespoons nutritional yeast

2 tablespoons red wine vinegar

2 teaspoons sea salt

½ teaspoon freshly ground black pepper

½ teaspoon onion powder

¼ teaspoon garlic powder

¼ teaspoon dried tarragon

For the salad

⅓ cup Garlic-Herb Bread Crumbs (page 127)

1 small head iceberg lettuce, cored and quartered into wedges

¼ cup cooked and crumbled uncured bacon

1 cup halved cherry tomatoes

1 small shallot, thinly sliced into rings

1 tablespoon chopped chives

1. Make the mayo and bread crumbs.

2. **Make the dressing.** In a medium mixing bowl, combine the mayo, nutritional yeast, red wine vinegar, salt, black pepper, onion powder, garlic powder, and tarragon. Whisk until creamy.

3. **Make the salad.** Hold a quartered wedge of lettuce in your hands and gently bend it in half, tearing some of the layers in the process. Transfer it to a plate, laying it flat, and spoon 2 tablespoons dressing over it. Sprinkle the wedge with bacon, tomatoes, shallot, chives, and bread crumbs. Repeat with the remaining 3 wedges and serve immediately. Refrigerate the extra salad dressing in an airtight container for up to 1 month.

PER SERVING: *Calories: 316; Total fat: 28g; Sodium: 588mg; Carbohydrates: 12g; Fiber: 3g; Protein: 6g; Iron: 1mg*

Melon Salad with Beet Vinaigrette

» 30 Minutes, Vegetarian   » Serves 2   » Prep time: 20 minutes

There are over 20 types of melon, and within that category, over 50 varieties of watermelons alone. While there are many kinds of melons, they all share one quality: They contain collagen, which is responsible for maintaining cell structure in connective tissue and is associated with supporting healthy skin. Try using any type of melon you can find in this summery salad paired with a healthy beet vinaigrette.

For the dressing

1 cup shredded red beets
1 cup red wine vinegar
¼ cup honey
1 teaspoon sea salt
¼ teaspoon freshly ground
  black pepper
1 mint sprig
½ cup olive oil

For the salad

2 cups baby arugula
½ cup cantaloupe, cut into
  1-inch chunks
½ cup honeydew melon,
  cut into 1-inch chunks
1 cup watermelon, cut into
  1-inch chunks
1 small shallot, sliced thin
2 radishes, sliced thin

1. **Make the dressing.** Combine the beets, red wine vinegar, honey, salt, pepper, and mint in a blender. Blend on medium speed and slowly drizzle in the olive oil on medium speed. Continue blending for 30 seconds, or until fully incorporated.

2. **Make the salad.** In a medium bowl, combine the arugula, cantaloupe, honeydew, watermelon, shallot, and radishes and toss to combine. Add 3 tablespoons vinaigrette and stir gently to coat. Serve immediately and refrigerate the remaining beet vinaigrette in an airtight container for up to 2 weeks.

Make It Easier: You can find packages of precut melons in the produce section of most grocery stores. This will cut way down on prep time and is a good buy if you're worried you won't be able to use up whole melons before they spoil.

PER SERVING: *Calories: 174; Total fat: 9g; Sodium: 132mg; Carbohydrates: 22g; Fiber: 2g; Protein: 2g; Iron: 1mg*

Minty Fruit Salad

» One-Pot, 30 Minutes, Vegetarian

» Serves 4

» Prep time: 10 minutes, plus 1 hour to marinate

Fruit salad is a classic for backyard barbecues, pool parties, and summer afternoons. This elegant take on fruit salad features fresh mint, which has been shown to aid in digestion and even reduce cold and flu symptoms. Letting this salad marinate for at least 1 hour before serving ensures that the fruit has time to take on the aroma and flavors of the mint for maximum flavor.

1 cup strawberries, trimmed and halved

½ cup blueberries

½ cup pineapple, cut into 1-inch chunks

1 cup grapes

1 cup cantaloupe, cut into 1-inch chunks

1 tablespoon honey

Zest of 1 lime

¼ cup fresh orange juice

2 tablespoons finely chopped fresh mint leaves

In a medium bowl, combine the strawberries, blueberries, pineapple, grapes, cantaloupe, honey, lime zest, orange juice, and mint. Refrigerate for at least 1 hour prior to serving. Keep leftovers refrigerated in an airtight container for up to 3 days.

Ingredient Swaps: You can make this recipe with almost any fruit, so tailor it to your personal preferences—try using honeydew in place of cantaloupe and blackberries in place of grapes. Do avoid bananas, as they tend to get mushy quickly when used in fruit salads and may not hold up as well as the rest of the fruit.

PER SERVING: *Calories: 97; Total fat: 0g; Sodium: 9mg; Carbohydrates: 25g; Fiber: 2g; Protein: 1g; Iron: 1mg*

Winter Squash Salad with Spiced Maple Vinaigrette

» 30 Minutes, Vegetarian   » Serves 2   » Prep time: 10 minutes
Cook time: 20 minutes

Winter squash is actually first harvested in the fall, but it stays in season through the winter months. Some of the most common winter squashes are delicata, acorn, butternut, Hubbard, spaghetti, and turban squash. You can use almost any winter squash in this recipe, but we use butternut and delicata for their thick flesh. Roasting the squash brings out its natural sweetness, making it a perfect complement to the smoky paprika in the Spiced Maple Vinaigrette (page 154).

For the squash

1 small butternut squash,
   peeled, deseeded
   and cubed
1 small delicata squash,
   deseeded and sliced into
   ½-inch pieces
1 tablespoon olive oil
1 teaspoon sea salt
½ teaspoon freshly ground
   black pepper

For the salad

2 tablespoons Spiced
   Maple Vinaigrette
   (page 154)
2 cups baby spinach
2 cups baby kale
3 tablespoons toasted
   pumpkin seeds

1. Preheat the oven to 400°F.

2. In a medium mixing bowl, combine the butternut and delicata squash and toss with the olive oil, salt, and pepper. Transfer the squash to a 9-by-13-inch baking dish and roast for 20 minutes, until tender and slightly golden brown. Remove the squash from the oven and set aside to cool.

3. While the squash cools, make the vinaigrette.

4. **Make the salad.** Combine the baby spinach and baby kale and divide between two plates. Top the greens with the roasted squash and pumpkin seeds, then drizzle each plate with 1 tablespoon vinaigrette. Serve immediately.

Make It Easier: Most winter squashes have an inedible rind, meaning they must be peeled prior to cutting and cooking. Delicata squash, however, has a thin rind that is edible. If you're short on time, use delicata to cut down on prep time.

PER SERVING: *Calories: 401; Total fat: 19g; Sodium: 659mg; Carbohydrates: 62g; Fiber: 11g; Protein: 9g; Iron: 5mg*

Shaved Brussels Sprouts Salad with Dried Cranberries

» 30 Minutes, Vegetarian, Low-Carb

» Serves 2

» Prep time: 20 minutes

Brussels sprouts are loaded with vitamin C, as well as the natural inflammation-reducing flavonoid kaempferol. The slight bitterness of the sprouts is well balanced in this salad with sweet apples and almonds and a lemony cranberry-mustard dressing.

For the dressing

¼ cup lemon juice

2 tablespoons cranberry juice

2 tablespoons Dijon mustard

1 tablespoon honey

1 teaspoon sea salt

½ teaspoon freshly ground black pepper

¾ cup olive oil

For the salad

3 cups Brussels sprouts, halved and thinly sliced

1 small Granny Smith apple, thinly sliced

1 large shallot, thinly sliced

½ cup unsweetened dried cranberries

⅓ cup toasted slivered almonds

1. **Make the dressing.** In a blender, combine the lemon juice, cranberry juice, mustard, honey, salt, and pepper. Blend on medium speed and slowly drizzle in the olive oil in an even stream. Continue blending until emulsified—the dressing should appear creamy.

2. **Make the salad.** In a medium bowl, combine the Brussels sprouts, apple, and shallot and toss. Divide the Brussels sprouts salad between two plates. Drizzle each serving with 2 tablespoons dressing and top with cranberries and toasted almonds. Serve immediately and refrigerate the extra dressing in an airtight container for up to 2 weeks.

Make It Easier: Many grocery stores, such as Sprouts and Whole Foods, sell packaged pre-shaved Brussels sprouts. Pick up a bag to make preparation for this recipe quick and easy.

PER SERVING: *Calories: 455; Total fat: 26g; Sodium: 186mg; Carbohydrates: 54g; Fiber: 11g; Protein: 9g; Iron: 3mg*

Parsnip "Potato" Salad

» 30 Minutes, Vegetarian   » Serves 2   » Prep time:10 minutes
                                          Cook time: 25 minutes

Parsnips are extremely hearty and high in fiber and have the same starchy texture as potatoes without a high glycemic index. In this recipe, we use parsnips instead of potatoes for a healthier spin on the traditional Southern potato salad. The rendered bacon fat is key to dressing the potato salad—that's what gives this recipe its rich flavor.

1 pound parsnips,
   peeled and cut into
   1-inch chunks
3 quarts water
6 slices uncured bacon
¼ cup apple cider vinegar
¼ cup Dijon mustard
1 tablespoon chopped
   scallions
1 small shallot, diced
1 teaspoon sea salt
½ teaspoon freshly ground
   black pepper

1. In a medium pot, bring the parsnips to a boil in the water. Continue cooking until the parsnips are tender, about 15 minutes. Drain the parsnips and set them aside to cool.

2. In a medium sauté pan, cook the bacon for 4 minutes on each side, until the fat is rendered. Set the bacon aside for use in a different recipe.

3. In a blender, combine the rendered bacon fat, apple cider vinegar, and mustard. Blend on medium speed until smooth.

4. Transfer the cooled parsnips to a medium bowl. Add the scallions, shallot, salt, and pepper. Pour in the bacon fat mixture and toss to coat. Serve immediately or refrigerate in an airtight container for up to 3 days.

Make It Easier: You can cook the parsnips up to 3 days in advance for faster preparation. Keep them refrigerated in an airtight container until you're ready to use them. You can also freeze raw parsnips for later use without damaging their flavor or texture.

PER SERVING: *Calories: 341; Total fat: 12g; Sodium: 1483mg; Carbohydrates: 47g; Fiber: 13g; Protein: 13g; Iron: 2mg*

Mediterranean-Style Steak Salad

» Low-Carb,
Diabetes-Friendly

» Serves 2

» Prep time: 15 minutes
Cook time: 20 minutes

This hearty but refreshing steak salad recipe is Paleo-friendly and also in line with the Mediterranean diet, featuring a medley of vegetables, lean steak, and a rich dressing full of healthy fats. Try using the dressing as a marinade for Grilled Flank Steak (page 109).

For the dressing

1 cup Paleo Mayo
(page 156)
¼ cup balsamic vinegar
1 tablespoon minced garlic
½ teaspoon dried oregano
1 teaspoon sea salt
½ teaspoon freshly ground
black pepper

For the salad

1 pound flank steak
1 tablespoon olive oil
4 cups mixed greens
1 small red bell pepper, cut
into ¼-inch strips
½ small red onion,
thinly sliced
½ English cucumber,
sliced into ¼-inch rounds
1 large beefsteak tomato,
cut into wedges
⅓ cup sliced black olives
2 teaspoons chopped fresh
mint leaves, for garnish

1. Make the mayo.

2. **Make the dressing.** In a medium bowl, combine the mayo, balsamic vinegar, garlic, oregano, salt, and pepper. Whisk vigorously until thoroughly combined. Reserve 2 tablespoons as a marinade for the steak.

3. Clean and trim the flank steak. Once that's done, place it in a shallow dish. Rub 2 tablespoons of the dressing onto the steak and marinate for 10 minutes.

4. Heat the olive oil in a large sauté pan over medium-high heat. Sear the flank steak for 4 to 5 minutes on each side, then remove from heat. Cover it with aluminum foil and let it rest for 5 minutes.

5. **Make the salad.** In a large bowl, combine the mixed greens, bell pepper, onion, cucumber, tomato, and olives. Add 2 tablespoons dressing and gently toss to coat. Transfer the dressed salad to two plates.

6. Cut the steak into ½-inch strips, slicing against the grain. Layer the steak on top of the salad and garnish with fresh mint. Refrigerate the extra dressing in an airtight container for up to 2 weeks.

PER SERVING: *Calories: 522; Total fat: 42g; Sodium: 421mg; Carbohydrates: 14g; Fiber: 5g; Protein: 52g; Iron: 6mg*

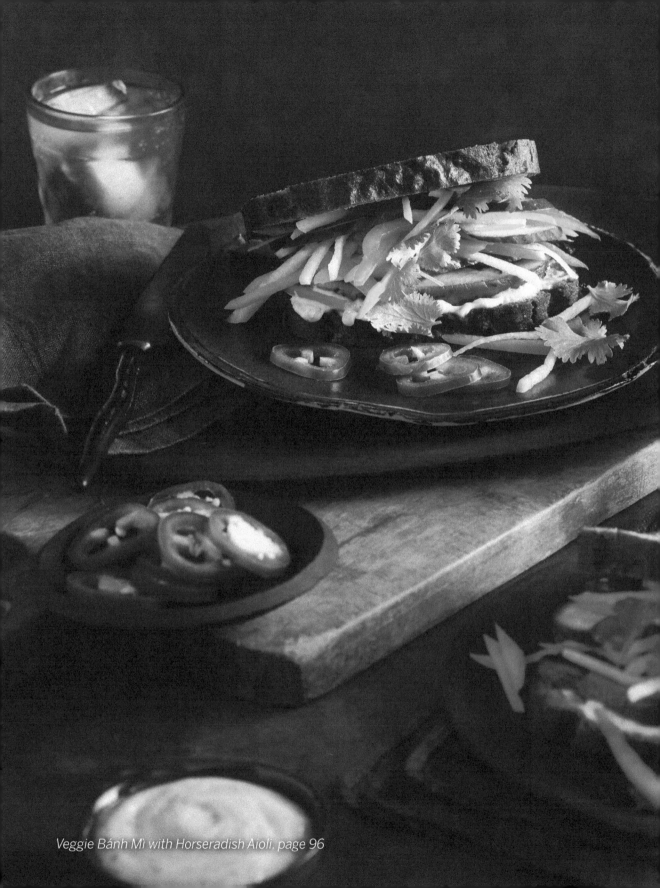

Veggie Bánh Mì with Horseradish Aioli, page 96

CHAPTER SIX

Soups and Sandwiches

— ◇ —

Soups and sandwiches are both lunchtime staples. When you first switch to the Paleo diet, you may worry that you will no longer be able to enjoy them, since many sandwiches use bread and cheese and many soups use cream. In reading this chapter, you'll see that you can still enjoy soups and sandwiches across the flavor spectrum. Just as salads are generally thought of as a summer dish, soups are often considered dishes to eat only during the winter. We turn this assumption on its head with refreshing summer soup recipes, such as Watermelon and Peach Gazpacho (page 81) and Roasted Tomato and Peach Soup with Strawberry Salsa (page 82).

A note: Our sandwich recipes all use our Paleo-friendly Almond Meal Sandwich Bread (page 121). We recommend keeping a loaf or two of this on hand so you can have it ready to prepare sandwiches.

Watermelon and Peach Gazpacho

» Low-Carb, Vegetarian   » Serves 2   » Prep time: 20 minutes, plus 1 hour to chill

Gazpacho is a chilled soup from Spain, traditionally composed of raw vegetables and herbs pureed with a tomato base. In this recipe, we add fresh fruit for a summery twist. This recipe has both a blended soup base and a chopped topping, but don't be overwhelmed by the ingredient list—many of the ingredients are used in both components.

For the soup

2 cups coarsely chopped
   ripe tomatoes
2 cups cubed watermelon
1 red bell pepper,
   coarsely chopped
½ English cucumber,
   coarsely chopped
½ small jalapeño,
   coarsely chopped
¼ cup sherry vinegar
1 tablespoon sea salt

For the topping

½ cup halved cherry
   tomatoes
1 cup finely diced
   watermelon
½ English cucumber,
   peeled and finely diced
½ small jalapeño,
   finely diced
1 ripe peach, pitted and
   finely diced
¼ cup finely diced
   red onion

2 tablespoons olive oil
Zest and juice of 1 lime
2 teaspoons sea salt
1 teaspoon freshly ground
   black pepper

For serving

2 tablespoons chopped
   fresh mint, for garnish
2 tablespoons chopped
   fresh basil, for garnish
2 tablespoons chopped
   cilantro, for garnish

1. **Make the soup.** In a blender, combine the tomatoes, watermelon, bell pepper, cucumber, jalapeño, sherry vinegar, and salt. Blend on high for 3 minutes, then chill in the refrigerator for 1 hour.

2. **Make the topping.** In a medium bowl, combine the cherry tomatoes, watermelon, English cucumber, jalapeño, peach, red onion, olive oil, lime zest and juice, salt, and pepper. Stir gently to combine; then chill in the refrigerator for 1 hour.

3. Chill two soup bowls in preparation for serving. When ready to serve, ladle the soup into the bowls and spoon the topping over it. Garnish with mint, basil, and cilantro.

PER SERVING: *Calories: 319; Total fat: 15g; Sodium: 2930mg; Carbohydrates: 45g; Fiber: 7g; Protein: 6g; Iron: 2mg*

Roasted Tomato and Peach Soup with Strawberry Salsa

» Low-Carb, Vegetarian   » Serves 4   » Prep time: 20 minutes
                                            Cook time: 20 minutes

This roasted tomato soup is one of our summertime favorites, and it's super healthy. It's also easy to make—just toss the vegetables on a baking sheet, roast, and then blend. Enjoy this salsa-topped soup served hot or chilled.

For the salsa

1 cup diced fresh
  strawberries
1 small jalapeño,
  finely diced
½ small red
  onion, chopped
2 tablespoons chopped
  fresh basil
1 tablespoon chopped
  fresh mint

1 tablespoon lime juice
2 teaspoons honey
1 teaspoon sea salt
¼ teaspoon freshly ground
  black pepper

For the soup

2 pounds Roma toma-
  toes, halved
1 pound peaches, halved
  and pitted

1 small onion, halved
2 tablespoons olive oil
4 cups vegetable stock
1 tablespoon sea salt
2 teaspoons freshly ground
  black pepper

1. Preheat the oven to 450°F and line a large baking sheet with parchment paper.

2. **Make the salsa.** In a medium bowl, combine the strawberries, jalapeño, red onion, basil, mint, lime juice, honey, salt, and pepper. Mix gently to combine, being careful to avoid mashing the strawberries. Chill in the refrigerator for 30 minutes while you make the soup.

3. **Make the soup.** Toss the tomatoes, peaches, and onion with the olive oil directly on the baking sheet. Roast for 15 to 20 minutes, or until the onion begins to brown. Transfer the roasted vegetables to a blender and add the stock, salt, and pepper. Blend on medium speed for 3 minutes, until smooth. Alternatively, combine all the ingredients in a bowl and blend with an immersion blender.

4. Ladle the soup into bowls and top with the chilled strawberry salsa. Refrigerate left-over soup and salsa in separate airtight containers for up to 3 days.

PER SERVING: *Calories: 183; Total fat: 8g; Sodium: 1726mg; Carbohydrates: 32g; Fiber: 6g; Protein: 4g; Iron: 1mg*

Avocado, Chicken, and Tarragon Salad Sandwich

» One-Pot, 30 Minutes, 5-Ingredient, Low-Carb, Diabetes-Friendly

» Serves 2

» Prep time: 20 minutes

We use avocado in place of mayonnaise in this heart-healthy chicken salad recipe. Avocados do not begin to ripen until after they are picked, so if you place them in the refrigerator just after buying, you can significantly slow down the ripening process. If your avocados are hard and bright green, you can speed up the ripening process by placing them in a brown paper bag on the counter for a day or two.

2 ripe avocados

1 tablespoon dried tarragon

Zest and juice of ½ lemon

½ teaspoon sea salt

¼ teaspoon white pepper

½ pound chicken, cooked and small diced

4 slices Almond Meal Sandwich Bread (page 121)

1. Cut the avocados in half, remove the pits, and use a spoon to scrape the flesh into a medium bowl.

2. Add the tarragon, lemon zest and juice, salt, and white pepper to the bowl. Using a fork or pastry cutter, mash the avocados with the other ingredients until the mixture is smooth.

3. Add the chicken to the bowl and stir to incorporate.

4. To assemble sandwiches, spread half the chicken salad on a slice of Almond Meal Sandwich Bread and top with a second slice. Repeat for the second sandwich and serve immediately. Refrigerate leftover chicken salad for up to 3 days in an airtight container.

Scale It Up: Double this recipe for use on more sandwiches or to serve as a side with Everything Seed Crackers (page 55). To prevent the avocado from oxidizing and browning, cover leftovers with a layer of plastic wrap, pressing it down to remove any air pockets.

PER SERVING: *Calories: 1305; Total fat: 112g; Sodium: 950mg; Carbohydrates: 39g; Fiber: 22g; Protein: 46g; Iron: 6mg*

Chicken and Shrimp Gumbo

» Low-Carb,
Diabetes-Friendly

» Serves 4

» Prep time: 20 minutes
Cook time: 5 hours

Gumbo is the official state dish of Louisiana, but as with many regional dishes, there is great debate over how it should be prepared. Across the board, gumbo is cooked low and slow, with a rich stock, a meat, a thickener, and the Holy Trinity of Cajun cooking: celery, bell peppers, and onions. This recipe is based on Ashley's family recipe and uses a roux thickener as well as gumbo filé, a spice made from ground sassafras leaves.

½ cup avocado oil

1 cup almond flour or
   blanched almond meal

1 large yellow onion,
   finely diced

½ cup finely diced celery

½ cup finely diced green
   bell pepper

¼ cup finely diced scallions

¼ cup dried parsley

8 cups hot water

2 pounds boneless, skin-
   less chicken thighs

1 tablespoon olive oil

1 teaspoon sea salt

½ teaspoon freshly ground
   black pepper

½ pound shrimp,
   peeled and deveined,
   tails removed

1 tablespoon filé powder

1. Preheat the oven to 400°F.

2. Heat the avocado oil in a large pot with a lid over medium heat until shimmering. Slowly add the almond flour to the oil, stirring constantly. Cook for 10 to 15 minutes over medium-low heat, stirring constantly. Unlike wheat flour, almond meal will not brown.

3. Add the onion, celery, bell pepper, scallions, and parsley to the roux and cook for 10 minutes, until the onion is soft and translucent.

4. Add the water to the pot, cover, and let simmer for 3 hours.

5. While the gumbo base is simmering, place the chicken thighs in a baking dish, drizzle them with the olive oil, and season them with salt and pepper. Roast at 400°F for 40 minutes, until the internal temperature reaches 165°F.

6. Once cooked, remove the chicken thighs from the oven, add them to the pot, and continue simmering.

7. After the gumbo base has simmered for 3 hours, add the shrimp to the pot and simmer, covered, for 30 more minutes.

8. Once the shrimp are cooked, remove the gumbo from the heat, stir in the filé powder, and serve immediately.

Ingredient Swaps: Ashley's family loves to prepare this dish with freshly shucked oysters instead of shrimp. Follow the same preparation instructions, using the same amount of oysters instead of shrimp.

PER SERVING: *Calories: 764; Total fat: 53g; Sodium: 567mg; Carbohydrates: 11g; Fiber: 4g; Protein: 63g; Iron: 4mg*

"Hot Chicken" Sandwich

» 30 Minutes

» Serves 2

» Prep time: 5 minutes
Cook time: 25 minutes

"Hot Chicken" originated in Nashville nearly 100 years ago. The story goes that in the early 1900s, Thornton Prince's lover served him super-spicy fried chicken as revenge after he cheated on her. She expected it to make him sick, but he loved the dish and ultimately opened a restaurant where he served it. This is our Paleo-friendly take on Nashville Hot Chicken.

For the chicken

2 (6-ounce) raw boneless, skinless chicken breasts or thighs
1 (13½-ounce) can full-fat coconut milk
2 cups tapioca starch
2 teaspoons sea salt
1 teaspoon freshly ground black pepper
1 teaspoon garlic powder
1 teaspoon onion powder
2 cups avocado oil, for frying
¼ cup Paleo-compliant hot sauce

For serving

4 slices Almond Meal Sandwich Bread (page 121), toasted
¼ cup Refrigerator Dill Pickles (page 49)

1. Preheat the oven to 400°F.

2. In a small bowl, soak the chicken breasts in the coconut milk for 5 minutes while you make the dredging mix.

3. To make the dredging mix, combine the tapioca starch, salt, pepper, garlic powder, and onion powder in a small bowl. Remove the chicken breasts from the coconut milk and dredge them in the dredging mixture, making sure to coat them fully.

4. Heat the avocado oil in a medium sauté pan over medium heat until it is shimmering, about 3 minutes. Carefully place the dredged chicken breasts in the oil. Fry them on one side for 5 minutes; then flip them and fry on the other side for 3 minutes. The chicken will not be cooked through—it will finish cooking in the oven.

5. Transfer the fried chicken to a baking dish and bake it in the oven for 15 to 20 minutes, until the internal temperature reads 165°F. Remove the chicken from the oven and toss it in the hot sauce.

6. Serve each chicken breast between two slices of toasted Almond Meal Sandwich Bread, topped with Refrigerator Dill Pickles.

Ingredient Swaps: Cut the chicken into bite-size pieces to make "hot chicken" nuggets—try serving them with our Guilt-Free Ranch Dressing (page 160) for the ultimate game-day snack.

PER SERVING: *Calories: 1750; Total fat: 111g; Sodium: 2133mg; Carbohydrates: 134g; Fiber: 10g; Protein: 54g; Iron: 12mg*

Curried Tomato Soup

» Vegetarian, Low-Carb, Diabetes-Friendly

» Serves 2

» Prep time: 15 minutes
Cook time: 30 minutes

The term "curry" carries many different meanings, varying by region and preparation. In many cases, curry refers to vegetables or meat cooked in a spiced sauce. The yellow hue in many curry dishes comes from turmeric, which has been used for medicinal purposes in South Asia for thousands of years. Turmeric is usually found in grocery store "curry powder" spice blends. This "curried" soup uses a blend of spices cooked with coconut milk for a warm, hearty finish.

¼ cup olive oil

1 medium yellow onion, chopped

1 tablespoon minced garlic

2 tablespoons fresh ginger, grated

1 teaspoon coriander

2 tablespoons curry powder

¼ teaspoon red pepper flakes

2 cups chopped tomatoes

1 cup water

⅓ cup chopped cilantro

2 teaspoons sea salt

1 teaspoon freshly ground black pepper

2 cups full-fat coconut milk

1. Heat the olive oil in a pot over medium-low heat. Add the onion and cook for 8 to 10 minutes, until translucent and lightly golden.

2. Add the garlic, ginger, coriander, curry powder, and red pepper flakes. Continue cooking, stirring often, for 3 minutes, or until fragrant and aromatic.

3. Add the tomatoes, water, cilantro, salt, pepper, and coconut milk to the pot and bring the mixture to a boil. Once boiling, reduce the heat to a simmer and cook for 10 to 15 minutes.

4. Transfer the mixture to a blender and blend on medium speed for 2 minutes, or until smooth. Alternatively, use an immersion blender to blend the soup directly in the pot. Serve hot and refrigerate any leftovers for up to 5 days.

Scale It Up: This is a great recipe to double or triple for a crowd or to have leftovers to enjoy all week. To serve leftovers, reheat the soup in a pot over medium heat, stirring often, until it reaches a simmer.

PER SERVING: *Calories: 771; Total fat: 77g; Sodium: 1210mg; Carbohydrates: 25g; Fiber: 7g; Protein: 8g; Iron: 10mg*

Creamy Cauliflower Bisque with Old Bay–Infused Oil

» Low-Carb, Diabetes-Friendly

» Serves 2

» Prep time: 10 minutes
Cook time: 45 minutes

Infused oils are a quick and easy way to add sophisticated flavor and color to any dish. In this recipe, we use hot infusion to make Old Bay–infused oil, which complements the creamy blended cauliflower soup.

For the infused oil

⅛ cup olive oil
1 teaspoon Old Bay seasoning

For the soup

2 tablespoons olive oil
1 medium yellow onion, coarsely chopped
1 tablespoon minced garlic
3 cups chicken or vegetable stock
2 cups full-fat coconut milk
1 large head cauliflower, florets coarsely chopped
1 tablespoon fresh thyme leaves, chopped
2 teaspoons sea salt
1 teaspoon freshly ground black pepper

1. **Make the infused oil.** Heat the ⅛ cup olive oil and Old Bay in a small sauté pan over low heat for 10 to 12 minutes, until fragrant. Remove from the heat and set aside.

2. Heat the 2 tablespoons of olive oil in a large soup pot over medium heat. Add the onion and cook until translucent and lightly golden, about 8 minutes. Add the garlic and cook for 30 seconds. Add the stock, coconut milk, cauliflower, thyme, salt, and pepper and bring the mixture to a boil. Reduce the heat to low and simmer until the cauliflower is tender and almost falling apart, about 20 minutes.

3. Transfer the mixture to a blender and blend on medium speed, until smooth and creamy. Alternatively, use an immersion blender to blend the soup directly in the pot.

4. Serve the soup in two bowls garnished with the infused oil. Serve hot and refrigerate leftover soup for up to 5 days.

PER SERVING: *Calories: 841; Total fat: 77g; Sodium: 1412mg; Carbohydrates: 39g; Fiber: 10g; Protein: 14g; Iron: 9mg*

Shrimp Po'Boy

» 30 Minutes

» Serves 2

» Prep time: 25 minutes
Cook time: 5 minutes

Po'boy sandwiches emerged around New Orleans during the late 1800s. One origin legend says that the sandwich was created in a New Orleans restaurant owned by former streetcar conductors. The story goes that during a streetcar company strike, the owners promised to serve free sandwiches to out-of-work employees—the "poor boys." With the local accent, this became "po'boy." This is our Paleo ode to a time-honored favorite.

For the shrimp

1 cup tapioca flour, divided
1 large egg
1 tablespoon water
¼ cup almond flour or blanched almond meal
1 tablespoon paprika
2 teaspoons cayenne pepper

1 tablespoon plus ½ teaspoon sea salt, divided
½ pound (about 24) shrimp, peeled and deveined, tails removed
¼ cup olive oil

For serving

¼ cup Russian Dressing (page 94)
4 slices Almond Meal Sandwich Bread (page 121), toasted
1 cup shredded iceberg lettuce
1 tomato, cut into ¼-inch rounds

1. Prepare the dressing.

2. **Make the dredging mixtures.** Place ½ cup tapioca flour in a small bowl. In a second small bowl, whisk together the egg and water. In a third small bowl, thoroughly mix the remaining ½ cup tapioca flour, the almond flour, paprika, cayenne pepper, and 1 tablespoon salt.

3. Dredge the shrimp by dipping them first in the tapioca bowl, then in the egg mixture and finally in the seasoned almond and tapioca flour mixture, pressing gently so it sticks. Repeat this process with all of the shrimp.

4. Heat the olive oil in a large sauté or cast-iron pan over medium-high heat until shimmering. Gently add the shrimp and cook for 2 to 4 minutes, turning halfway through, until golden and crispy. Work in batches to avoid overcrowding the pan.

5. Transfer the fried shrimp to a wire cooling rack and sprinkle them with the remaining ½ teaspoon salt.

6. **Assemble the sandwiches.** Spread both sides of the Almond Meal Sandwich Bread with dressing and top with shrimp, iceberg lettuce, and tomato slices. Serve immediately.

Ingredient Swaps: Po'boys are also made in New Orleans with fried oysters. Try using raw oysters in place of shrimp, prepared the same way, for a slightly stronger seafood flavor.

PER SERVING: *Calories: 792; Total fat: 72g; Sodium: 981mg; Carbohydrates: 34g; Fiber: 7g; Protein: 27g; Iron: 5mg*

BBQ Pulled Pork Sandwich

» Low-Carb,
Diabetes-Friendly

» Serves 4

» Prep time: 5 minutes
Cook time: 6 hours

There are four main styles of barbecue sauces—Memphis, Carolina, Kansas City, and Texas—each delicious in their own way. We serve this slow-roasted pulled pork recipe with BBQ Sauce (page 158), which combines Memphis-style and Kansas City–style sauces for a touch of sweetness and a subtle smoky flavor.

For the pulled pork

2 pounds boneless
   pork loin
3 cups apple cider vinegar
1 tablespoon chipo-
   tle peppers
1 tablespoon mustard
   powder
1 tablespoon smoked
   paprika
1 (6-ounce) can
   tomato paste
2 tablespoons sea salt
2 tablespoons freshly
   ground black pepper

For serving

½ cup BBQ Sauce
   (page 158)
½ cup Creamy Kale Slaw
   (page 50)
4 slices Almond Meal
   Sandwich Bread
   (page 121)

1. Preheat the oven to 250°F and place the pork loin in a deep baking dish.

2. In a medium bowl, combine the apple cider vinegar, chipotle peppers, mustard powder, smoked paprika, tomato paste, salt, and pepper. Whisk to combine.

3. Pour the marinade over the pork. Cover the baking dish tightly with two layers of aluminum foil. Place the pork roast in the oven and let it roast for 6 hours.

4. While the pork loin cooks, prepare the BBQ sauce and slaw.

5. After cooking, remove the dish from the oven and let it cool for 15 minutes. Use two forks to shred the pork. Dress the pulled pork with sauce and serve between two slices of Almond Meal Sandwich Bread topped with slaw, with extra sauce on the side.

Ingredient Swaps: Try skipping the bread and instead serve the pulled pork over a baked sweet potato, topped with fresh cilantro and barbecue sauce. It's a great way to use up any extra meat leftovers.

PER SERVING: *Calories: 734; Total fat: 40g; Sodium: 2215mg; Carbohydrates: 28g; Fiber: 7g; Protein: 60g; Iron: 5mg*

Butternut Squash Soup

» One-Pot, Low-Carb, Diabetes-Friendly

» Serves 2

» Prep time: 10 minutes
Cook time: 40 min

Butternut squash, a hardy winter squash, has a thick skin that gives it a long shelf life. Its skin is not edible, so use a vegetable peeler to peel it before coring and slicing it for this recipe. Butternut squash is ideal for Paleo cooking—it is rich in complex carbohydrates, high in fiber, and naturally sweet but with a low glycemic index. In this one-pot recipe, we blend the squash with coconut milk to create a rich, creamy soup.

2 tablespoons olive oil

½ small yellow onion, coarsely chopped

2 tablespoons minced garlic

3 cups cubed butternut squash, peeled and cored

1½ cups full-fat coconut milk

1½ cups chicken or vegetable stock

2 tablespoons maple syrup

2 teaspoons chopped fresh thyme leaves, plus more for garnish

2 teaspoons curry powder

¼ teaspoon ground cinnamon

2 teaspoons sea salt

1 teaspoon freshly ground black pepper

1. Heat the olive oil in a large soup pot over medium-low heat. Add the onion and cook, stirring occasionally, for 12 to 15 minutes, until the onion is golden brown and slightly caramelized. Add the garlic and cook for 1 minute, stirring occasionally.

2. Add the butternut squash, coconut milk, stock, maple syrup, thyme leaves, curry powder, cinnamon, salt, and pepper. Bring the mixture to a boil, then reduce the heat to low and simmer for 25 minutes, until the squash is tender.

3. Transfer the mixture to a blender and blend to puree, about 3 minutes, or use an immersion blender to puree the soup directly in the pot. Garnish with additional thyme leaves and serve hot.

Make It Easier: Many grocery stores carry precut butternut squash—purchase a bag to cut the prep time of this dish in half.

PER SERVING: *Calories: 636; Total fat: 50g; Sodium: 1411mg; Carbohydrates: 51g; Fiber: 6g; Protein: 7g; Iron: 8mg*

Turkey Reuben Lettuce Wraps

» One-Pot, 30 Minutes, Low-Carb   » Serves 2   » Prep time: 15 minutes

A traditional Reuben is made with corned beef, Swiss cheese, sauerkraut, and Russian dressing between two slices of rye bread. Here, we've taken the original Reuben and turned it into a healthy spin-off, with turkey breast instead of corned beef and our own homemade Russian dressing. You can buy precooked turkey or cook boneless turkey breast at 375°F for about 20 minutes, until the internal temperature reaches 165°F.

For the Russian dressing

1 cup Paleo Mayo (page 156)
2 tablespoons horseradish
2 teaspoons coconut aminos
1 tablespoon coconut sugar
1 teaspoon paprika
1 teaspoon sea salt
½ teaspoon freshly ground black pepper
1 teaspoon Paleo-compliant hot sauce

For the wraps

4 Bibb lettuce leaves
10 ounces cooked turkey breast, sliced into ½-inch strips
½ cup Paleo-compliant sauerkraut (such as Wildbrine Raw Organic Sauerkraut)

1. Prepare the mayo.

2. **Make the dressing.** In a small bowl, combine the mayo, horseradish, coconut aminos, coconut sugar, paprika, salt, pepper, and hot sauce. Whisk until smooth.

3. **Assemble the wraps.** Fold the four lettuce leaves into cups. In each leaf, layer 2 tablespoons Russian dressing, one-quarter of the turkey, and ¼ cup sauerkraut. Serve immediately and store extra dressing for up to 5 days.

Scale It Up: This Russian dressing in this recipe can be used for almost any sandwich, including the Shrimp Po'Boy (page 90). Double the recipe and save it for use later in the week.

PER SERVING: *Calories: 446; Total fat: 30g; Sodium: 649mg; Carbohydrates: 2g; Fiber: 1g; Protein: 42g; Iron: 3mg*

Grilled Vegetable Sandwich with Mint Pesto

» 30 Minutes, Vegetarian, Low-Carb, Diabetes-Friendly

» Serves 2

» Prep time: 10 minutes
Cook time: 20 minutes

The vegetables in this recipe can be prepared on a grill or in a sauté pan. This recipe provides instructions for a sauté pan, but if the weather is nice, fire up the grill. Lightly dress the vegetables in olive oil and grill for about 5 minutes on each side. A quick tip: Be sure not to skip salting the eggplant—this is key to releasing some of its water and prevents it from getting soggy during cooking.

For the vegetables

1 tablespoon sea salt
1 small eggplant, cut into ½-inch rounds
1 tablespoon olive oil
1 small yellow summer squash, cut into ½-inch rounds
1 small zucchini, cut into ½-inch rounds
1 red bell pepper, cored and cut into 4 sections

For serving

¼ cup Nut-Free Pesto (page 157)
2 sprigs fresh mint, chopped
4 slices Almond Meal Sandwich Bread, toasted (page 121)

1. Generously salt the eggplant and allow it to rest for 20 minutes before cooking.

2. While the eggplant rests, prepare the pesto.

3. Heat the olive oil in a large sauté pan over medium heat. Add the yellow squash and zucchini to the pan in a single layer and cook for 3 minutes on each side, until they are tender and have a slight char. Remove the squash and zucchini, set aside, and repeat with the bell pepper and eggplant.

4. In a small bowl, combine the pesto and chopped mint. Stir to combine.

5. **Assemble the sandwiches.** Spread 1 tablespoon mint pesto on a slice of Almond Meal Sandwich Bread. Top with the grilled vegetables and a second slice of bread. Serve immediately.

Scale It Up: Double the recipe for the grilled vegetables and serve them in a large dish (without bread) with mint pesto on the side. This makes a great appetizer for a group gathering.

PER SERVING: *Calories: 660; Total fat: 51g; Sodium: 1670mg; Carbohydrates: 39g; Fiber: 16g; Protein: 21g; Iron: 4mg*

Veggie Bánh Mì with Horseradish Aioli

» 30 Minutes

» Serves 2

» Prep time: 25 minutes
Cook time: 5 minutes

Bánh is the Vietnamese word for bread, and *bánh mì* is a Vietnamese sandwich usually served on a short baguette with meat and vegetables. In our version, we use pickled vegetables, which provide a generous dose of vitamins, minerals, and probiotics. We also add portabella mushrooms for rich umami flavor, satisfying to vegetarians and meat-lovers alike.

For the pickled vegetables

½ cup carrot, shredded

½ cup cucumber, thinly sliced

½ cup red bell pepper, julienned

½ cup daikon radish, shredded (optional)

2 tablespoons red wine vinegar

2 tablespoons coconut sugar

¼ teaspoon sea salt

For the bánh mì

2 large portabella mushrooms, cleaned and sliced into ½-inch strips

2 tablespoons fish sauce

2 tablespoons olive oil, divided

1 teaspoon coconut sugar

1 tablespoon minced garlic

4 slices Almond Meal Sandwich Bread, toasted (page 121), for serving

1 jalapeño, thinly sliced, for serving (optional)

¼ cup chopped fresh cilantro, for serving (optional)

For the aioli

1 cup Paleo Mayo (page 156)

¼ cup horseradish root, freshly grated

2 teaspoons Dijon mustard

1 teaspoon ground coriander (optional)

1 teaspoon sea salt

½ teaspoon freshly ground black pepper

1. **Prepare the pickled vegetables.** In a medium bowl, combine the carrots, cucumbers, bell pepper, daikon radish, red wine vinegar, 2 tablespoons coconut sugar, and salt. Toss the mixture several times and set aside to pickle for at least 20 minutes.

2. While the vegetables pickle, prepare the mayo.

3. In a small bowl, combine the mushrooms, fish sauce, 1 tablespoon olive oil, 1 teaspoon coconut sugar, and the minced garlic.

4. Heat the remaining 1 tablespoon olive oil in a large skillet over medium heat. Once the oil is shimmering, lay the mushroom pieces in the skillet and cook for 2 to 3 minutes, flipping halfway through. Remove from the heat and place on a paper towel.

5. **Prepare the aioli.** In a small bowl, combine the mayo, horseradish, mustard, coriander (if using), salt, and pepper. Whisk until fully incorporated.

6. Drain the pickled vegetables.

7. **Assemble the sandwiches.** Spread a thin layer of horseradish aioli on a slice of bread. Top with the mushrooms, pickled vegetables, jalapeño slices, and cilantro, if using. Top with a second slice of bread and serve immediately.

Make It Easier: To save time, prepare the pickled vegetables in advance—they will keep for up to 1 week in the refrigerator.

PER SERVING: *Calories: 705; Total fat: 61g; Sodium: 2070mg; Carbohydrates: 25g; Fiber: 8g; Protein: 20g; Iron: 4mg*

Waldorf-Style Chicken Salad Sandwich

» One-Pot, 30 Minutes   » Serves 2   » Prep time: 10 minutes

The chicken salad in this sandwich recipe is on the sweet-and-tart side, as a result of the natural sugars in the dried blueberries, apple, and grapes. Make sure to use unsweetened dried blueberries without added sugar. We serve this chicken salad on sandwiches, but it can also be served over a bed of lettuce, with Everything Seed Crackers (page 55), or on its own as a side.

1 pound cooked chicken breast, diced

½ cup Paleo Mayo (page 156)

½ cup halved seedless red grapes

¼ cup dried blueberries

1 small Granny Smith apple, diced

½ cup chopped pecans

¼ cup chopped celery

1 teaspoon coconut sugar

2 teaspoons sea salt

1 teaspoon freshly ground black pepper

4 slices Almond Meal Sandwich Bread (page 121), for serving

In a medium bowl, combine the chicken, mayo, grapes, dried blueberries, apple, pecans, celery, coconut sugar, salt, and pepper. Mix well to combine. Serve between two slices of sandwich bread. Refrigerate extra chicken salad in an airtight container for up to 3 days.

Scale It Up: This recipe makes a quick and easy on-the-go lunch—double the recipe to have leftovers to enjoy the next day.

PER SERVING: *Calories: 1492; Total fat: 111g; Sodium: 2024mg; Carbohydrates: 40g; Fiber: 11g; Protein: 89g; Iron: 6mg*

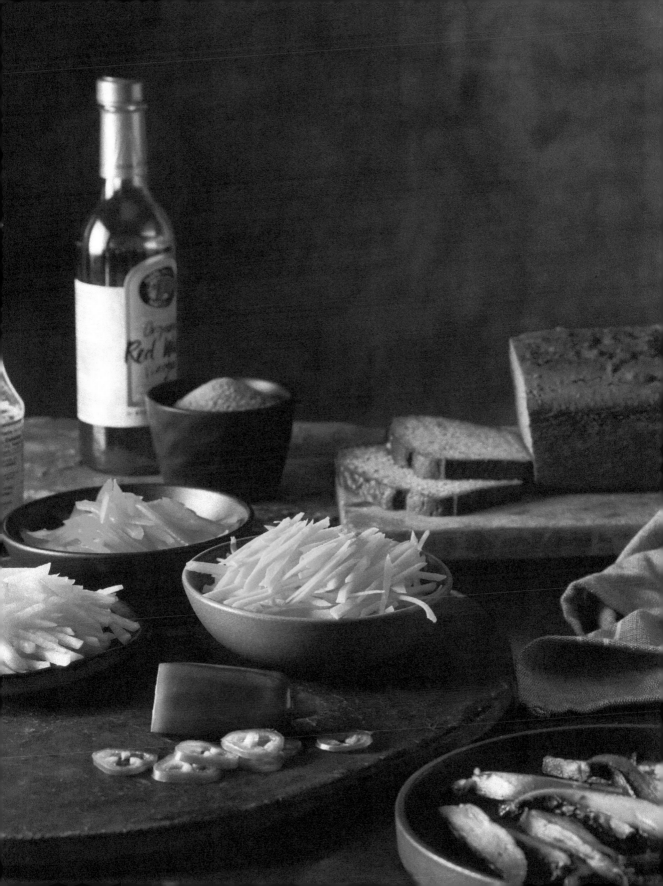

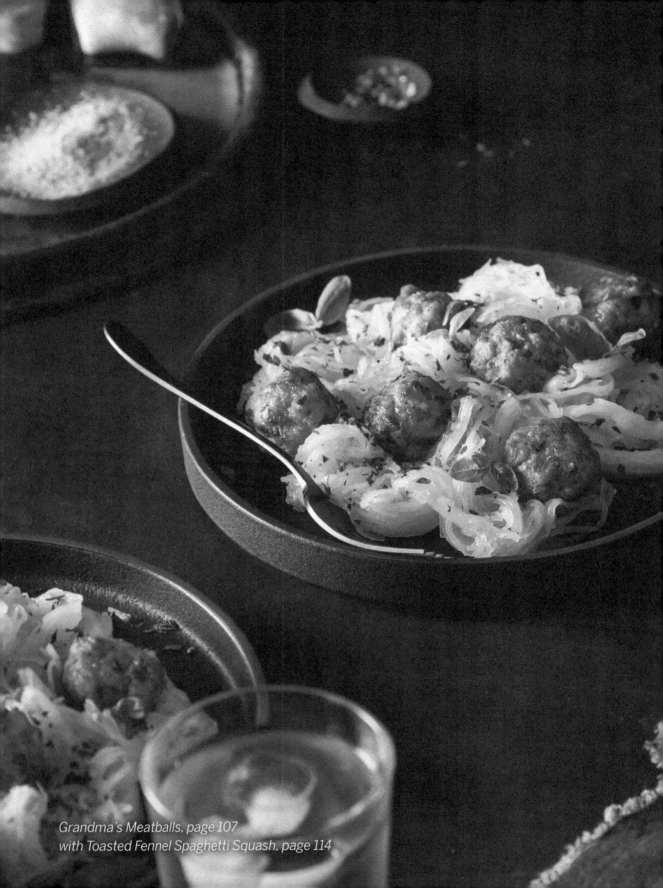

Grandma's Meatballs, page 107
with Toasted Fennel Spaghetti Squash, page 114

CHAPTER SEVEN

Mains

In this chapter, we present 15 main dish recipes to enjoy, and we recommend side dishes to pair with almost all of them for a complete meal. The recipes in this chapter cover a wide range of flavor profiles and cuisines, including American, Indian, Mexican, Chinese, Italian, and Korean. We encourage you to explore these recipes and discover new ingredients that you may not have cooked with or even heard of before. You may surprise yourself with the flavor combinations you enjoy, and you may gravitate toward cuisines you previously shied away from. Cooking for two provides a great opportunity to take a chance and try something new together.

Seared Mahi-Mahi with Coconut-Caper Sauce

» 30 Minutes, Low-Carb, Diabetes-Friendly

» Serves 2

» Prep time: 5 minutes
Cook time: 20 minutes

Mahi-mahi is a lean, mild whitefish that can be grilled, seared, fried, or baked. When preparing mahi-mahi, avoid overcooking it, which will cause the flesh to become dry and tough. Correctly cooked mahi-mahi should be opaque but still have a smooth, buttery texture. The light fish and coconut sauce in this dish will pair well with Cauliflower "Rice" (page 54) and Asparagus Amandine (page 57).

3 tablespoons olive oil, divided

2 teaspoons minced garlic

1 cup full-fat coconut milk

2 tablespoons drained capers

2 teaspoons freshly squeezed lemon juice

1½ teaspoons sea salt, divided

½ teaspoon freshly ground black pepper, divided

1 tablespoon chopped fresh parsley

2 (5- to 7-ounce) mahi-mahi fillets

1. **Make the sauce.** Heat 1 tablespoon olive oil in a medium sauté pan over medium heat. Add the garlic and cook for 2 minutes, until fragrant. Add the coconut milk and bring the mixture to a boil, then reduce the heat to low. Simmer for 3 minutes, until the sauce thickens.

2. Remove the sauce from heat and stir in the capers, lemon juice, ½ teaspoon salt, ¼ teaspoon pepper, and the parsley. Cover and set aside to keep warm.

3. Lightly pat the fillets with a paper towel to absorb any excess liquid; this will ensure an even sear. Season the fillets on one side with the remaining 1 teaspoon salt and ¼ teaspoon pepper.

4. Heat the remaining 2 tablespoons olive oil in a large sauté pan over medium heat. Add the fillets to the pan, seasoned-side down, and sear undisturbed for 5 minutes. Flip and continue cooking for 3 to 5 minutes, until the internal temperature reaches 137°F.

5. Remove the fillets from the heat and transfer them to two plates. Top with the coconut-caper sauce and serve immediately.

PER SERVING: *Calories: 546; Total fat: 47g; Sodium: 1164mg; Carbohydrates: 5g; Fiber: 0g; Protein: 32g; Iron: 5mg*

Tandoori-Style Chicken

» One-Pot, Low-Carb,
  Diabetes-Friendly

» Serves 2

» Prep time: 15 minutes
  Cook time: 40 minutes

Tandoori chicken is an Indian recipe that is traditionally made by marinating chicken in spiced yogurt and cooking it in a *tandoor*, a clay oven heated with wood or charcoal. In this recipe, we roast the chicken at a high temperature to recreate the heat of a tandoor, and we use coconut milk in place of yogurt to make this dish Paleo-friendly. This dish pairs well with sautéed vegetables, such as squash and zucchini, or with roasted sweet potatoes.

Olive oil cooking spray, for greasing the pan

2 tablespoons ground coriander

2 tablespoons garam masala

2 teaspoons ground ginger

½ teaspoon turmeric

½ teaspoon smoked paprika

2 teaspoons sea salt

1 (13½-ounce) can full-fat coconut milk

1 tablespoon freshly squeezed lemon juice

1 tablespoon minced garlic

2 ounces fresh cilantro, coarsely chopped

1 pound boneless, skinless chicken thighs

1. Preheat the oven to 400°F. Lightly coat a 9-by-13-inch baking sheet with olive oil cooking spray.

2. In a medium bowl, combine the coriander, garam masala, ginger, turmeric, paprika, and salt. Add the coconut milk, lemon juice, garlic, and cilantro and stir to combine.

3. Add the chicken thighs to the coconut milk and spices and toss to coat completely. Then, transfer the coated chicken to the baking sheet. Roast for 30 to 40 minutes, until the internal temperature of the chicken reaches 165°F. Remove from the oven and serve immediately.

Make It Easier: Prepare the coconut milk and spice mixture ahead and marinate the chicken in it for up to 2 days in the refrigerator or 2 weeks in the freezer. Defrost in the refrigerator before cooking to make this a quick and easy weeknight dish.

PER SERVING: *Calories: 691; Total fat: 51g; Sodium: 1420mg; Carbohydrates: 13g; Fiber: 4g; Protein: 50g; Iron: 10mg*

Ginger-Beef Stir-Fry

» 30 Minutes

» Serves 2

» Prep time: 15 minutes
Cook time: 15 minutes

Stir-frying is a versatile technique in Chinese cooking in which ingredients are cooked quickly in hot oil. Cooking quickly preserves vitamins and minerals in fresh vegetables. Stir-frying is traditionally done in a wok, but you can use a large sauté pan for this smaller recipe. Try pairing this rich, aromatic dish with Cauliflower "Rice" (page 54).

For the stir-fry sauce

½ cup chopped pineapple
½ cup coconut aminos
¼ cup orange juice
1 tablespoon freshly
 squeezed lime juice
½ cup honey
1 teaspoon ground ginger
1 tablespoon minced garlic
2 teaspoons sesame oil

1 tablespoon sea salt
½ teaspoon red
 pepper flakes
1 tablespoon tapioca starch
¼ cup cold water

For the vegetables

1 tablespoon olive oil
1 large carrot, cut into
 ½-inch rounds

1 small head broccoli, cut
 into florets
1 small red bell pepper,
 julienned
1 small yellow onion,
 julienned
1 pound flank steak,
 trimmed and sliced into
 ½-inch strips

1. **Make the stir-fry sauce.** In a blender, combine the pineapple, coconut aminos, orange juice, lime juice, honey, ginger, garlic, sesame oil, salt, red pepper flakes, tapioca starch, and water. Blend on high speed for 2 minutes and set aside.

2. Heat the olive oil in a large sauté pan over high heat. Add the carrot and cook for 5 minutes, then add the broccoli and cook for another 5 minutes. Add the bell pepper and onion and continue cooking for another 5 minutes. Remove the cooked vegetables from the pan and set aside.

3. Add the steak to the large sauté pan and sear on high heat, stirring constantly for about 3 minutes, or until browned on the edges. Return the vegetables to the pan and sauté for 5 minutes. Add the sauce to the pan and cook for 3 minutes, until thickened. Serve immediately.

PER SERVING: *Calories: 922; Total fat: 31g; Sodium: 3921mg; Carbohydrates: 107g; Fiber: 8g; Protein: 60g; Iron: 7mg*

Chipotle-Apple Pork Chops

» 30 Minutes

» Serves 2

» Prep time: 5 minutes
Cook time: 20 minutes

Chipotle peppers are actually made from jalapeños. At the end of their growing period, ripe green jalapeños turn red and start to dry out. These overripe peppers are harvested and then smoke-dried, becoming chipotle peppers. This sweet-and-spicy pork chop recipe uses chipotles in adobo sauce, which are available in the Mexican food section of most grocery stores.

1 cup Zesty Ketchup (page 162)

2 cups organic unsweetened applesauce

¼ cup honey

2 tablespoons chopped chipotle peppers in adobo sauce

1 teaspoon cumin

2 bone-in pork chops, about 6 to 8 ounces each

2 teaspoons sea salt

1 teaspoon freshly ground black pepper

2 tablespoons olive oil

1 tablespoon chopped cilantro, for garnish

1. Prepare the ketchup.

2. **Make the chipotle-apple sauce.** In a small bowl, whisk together the applesauce, ketchup, honey, chipotle peppers, and cumin.

3. Season the pork chops generously on both sides with salt and pepper. In a large sauté pan, heat the oil over medium-high heat. Place the pork chops in the pan and cook for 5 minutes on one side.

4. After 5 minutes, flip the pork chops, reduce the heat to low, and add three-quarters of the sauce. Allow the pork chops to simmer in the sauce for 7 to 10 minutes, depending on their size.

5. Remove the pan from the heat and allow the pork chops to rest for 10 minutes—they will continue cooking while they rest.

6. Once rested, transfer the pork chops to plates, and top with the remaining sauce. Garnish with cilantro and serve immediately.

Make It Easier: You can make the chipotle-apple sauce up to 1 week in advance, keeping it refrigerated in an airtight container.

PER SERVING: *Calories: 764; Total fat: 1298g; Sodium: 18mg; Carbohydrates: 91g; Fiber: 3g; Protein: 36g; Iron: 4mg*

Grandma's Meatballs

» Low-Carb, Diabetes-Friendly

» Serves 2

» Prep time: 15 minutes
Cook time: 20 minutes

This comfort-food meatball recipe brings back memories of childhood dinners, with classic seasonings like fennel, onion, and garlic. Try serving them tossed in BBQ Sauce (page 158), with zoodles, or with Toasted Fennel Spaghetti Squash (page 114). To make them kid-friendly, serve with Zesty Ketchup (page 162). This recipe uses both ground beef and pork, but you could also use lamb if you prefer.

½ cup Garlic-Herb Bread Crumbs (page 127)

¼ cup full-fat coconut milk

1 pound ground beef

½ pound ground pork

2 tablespoons minced garlic

1 tablespoon toasted fennel seeds, chopped

1 tablespoon onion powder

2 teaspoons sea salt

1 teaspoon freshly ground black pepper

½ teaspoon red pepper flakes (optional)

2 large eggs, beaten

¼ cup freshly chopped parsley

2 tablespoons olive oil

1. Preheat the oven to 350°F. While the oven preheats, prepare the bread crumbs.

2. In a small bowl, combine the bread crumbs and coconut milk. Stir to combine and let rest for 10 minutes.

3. In a large bowl, combine the ground beef, ground pork, garlic, fennel seeds, onion powder, salt, pepper, and red pepper flakes (if using). Gently fold in the soaked bread crumbs, eggs, and parsley, stirring until just combined. Overmixing will lead to dense meatballs.

4. Roll the mixture into 1-inch meatballs and set in a dish for easy access.

5. Heat the olive oil in a large sauté pan over medium heat. Sear the meatballs on all sides so they develop a crust, 3 to 5 minutes (they will not be fully cooked). Work in batches to avoid overcrowding the pan.

6. Place the seared meatballs in a 9-by-13-inch baking dish. Bake for 10 to 15 minutes, or until the internal temperature registers at least 155°F. Serve hot.

Make It Easier: Make a double batch of the meatball mixture and freeze uncooked meatballs in a freezer bag for up to 1 month.

PER SERVING: *Calories: 989; Total fat: 62g; Sodium: 1660mg; Carbohydrates: 29g; Fiber: 4g; Protein: 80g; Iron: 11mg*

Sheet Pan Chicken Bake

» One-Pot, Low-Carb, Diabetes-Friendly

» Serves 2

» Prep time: 5 minutes
Cook time: 40 minutes

This simple sheet-pan chicken dressed with a lemony marinade is made for those lazy nights when you simply can't bear to wash a big load of dishes. All of the ingredients go on a single sheet pan for roasting, and voilà: Dinner is served. See the Ingredient Swaps tip after the recipe for ideas of different proteins, vegetables, and spices to use.

2 tablespoons freshly squeezed lemon juice

2 tablespoons olive oil, divided

1 tablespoon red wine vinegar

1 tablespoon minced garlic

2 tablespoons dried oregano

1 tablespoon dried basil

⅛ teaspoon red pepper flakes

2 pounds boneless, skinless chicken thighs

2 teaspoons sea salt

¼ teaspoon freshly ground black pepper

1 pound Brussels sprouts, halved

2 medium bell peppers, cut into ½-inch strips

1 small red onion, cut into ½-inch strips

1. Preheat the oven to 400°F and line a large rimmed baking sheet with parchment paper.

2. In a small bowl, whisk together the lemon juice, 1 tablespoon olive oil, the red wine vinegar, garlic, oregano, basil, and red pepper flakes. Set aside.

3. Pat the chicken dry with paper towels, place it in the center of the baking sheet, and season with salt and pepper. Spread the Brussels sprouts, cut-side down, around the edges of the pan, surrounding the chicken. Roast for 15 minutes.

4. Remove the baking sheet from the oven and add the bell peppers and onion, as well as half of the lemon juice mixture. Return to the oven and roast for 15 to 20 minutes, until the Brussels sprouts are crispy and the peppers and onions are tender. The chicken should have an internal temperature of 165°F.

5. Remove the sheet pan from the oven and drizzle with the remaining lemon mixture. Allow to cool for 5 minutes before serving.

Ingredient Swaps: Try using flank steak or chicken thighs instead of breasts and switching up the seasonings—for example, replace the oregano and basil with a combination of cumin and coriander.

PER SERVING: *Calories: 828; Total fat: 33g; Sodium: 1658mg; Carbohydrates: 33g; Fiber: 12g; Protein: 99g; Iron: 8mg*

Grilled Flank Steak with Zesty Mustard Sauce

» 30 Minutes, Low-Carb   » Serves 2   » Prep time: 15 minutes
Cook time: 10 minutes

When cooked properly, flank steak can be tender and flavorful. The key to a tender flank steak is avoiding overcooking it, so it should be prepared medium or medium-rare rather than well-done. Add moisture by serving it with a sauce, like the tangy mustard one in this recipe. When serving, flank steak should be sliced against the grain.

For the sauce

¼ cup coconut aminos
¼ cup stone-ground mustard
1 tablespoon coconut sugar
1 tablespoon fresh chopped thyme leaves
1 teaspoon red pepper flakes
1 teaspoon sea salt
1 teaspoon freshly ground black pepper

For the steak

1 pound flank steak, cleaned and cut in half
2 teaspoons sea salt, divided
2 tablespoons olive oil
1 teaspoon freshly ground black pepper

1. Place the flank steak on a wire rack and allow it to rest for 10 minutes at room temperature before cooking.

2. While the steak rests, make the mustard sauce. In a small bowl, whisk together the coconut aminos, mustard, coconut sugar, thyme, red pepper flakes, salt, and pepper. Set aside to chill in the refrigerator.

3. Once rested, pat the steak with paper towels to remove any excess moisture, then season it with 1 teaspoon salt.

4. Heat the olive oil in a large sauté or cast-iron pan over medium-high heat. Add the steak to the pan, pressing down on it with a spatula to ensure even contact. Sear undisturbed on one side for 3 to 4 minutes, then flip and sear for 3 to 4 more minutes.

5. Transfer the steak to a cutting board, cover, and let rest for 10 minutes. Then, cut the steak against the grain into ½-inch slices and season with the remaining 1 teaspoon of salt and the pepper.

6. Transfer the steak to two plates, drizzle with the mustard sauce, and serve immediately. Refrigerate extra sauce for up to 2 weeks.

PER SERVING: *Calories: 557; Total fat: 33g; Sodium: 2963mg; Carbohydrates: 10g; Fiber: 2g; Protein: 52g; Iron: 5mg*

Pesto Salmon

» 30 Minutes, Low-Carb,
Diabetes-Friendly

» Serves 2

» Prep time: 5 minutes
Cook time: 10 minutes

Wild-caught salmon is a fantastic source of omega-3 fatty acids. This super-healthy sautéed salmon is served with a pesto made with basil and spinach, which provide vitamins K, A, and C. We replace the Parmesan cheese normally used in pesto with nutritional yeast, which provides a cheesy flavor. We recommend pairing this dish with Asparagus Amandine (page 57).

2 cups fresh basil leaves

1 cup baby spinach leaves

½ cup plus 1 tablespoon olive oil, divided

¼ cup toasted pine nuts

1 tablespoon nutritional yeast

1 tablespoon minced garlic

½ teaspoon sea salt

¼ teaspoon white pepper

1 pound wild-caught salmon fillet, cut into two portions

1. **Make the pesto.** In the bowl of a food processor or blender, combine the basil, spinach, ½ cup olive oil, the pine nuts, nutritional yeast, garlic, salt, and white pepper. Pulse or blend on medium speed for 2 minutes, stopping to scrape down the sides with a spatula. The pesto should have a paste-like consistency. Transfer the pesto to a bowl and set aside.

2. Heat the remaining 1 tablespoon olive oil in a medium sauté pan over medium-high heat for 1 minute. Add the salmon to the pan and cook on one side for 3 to 4 minutes, depending on the size of your fillets. Flip and cook for an additional 2 to 3 minutes. The salmon should reach an internal temperature of 125°F. Remove from the heat.

3. Serve the salmon immediately, topped with the pesto.

Ingredient Swaps: Pine nuts are tasty but are also very expensive. If you don't have pine nuts on hand, substitute the same amount of walnuts or toasted sunflower seeds.

PER SERVING: *Calories: 473; Total fat: 28g; Sodium: 582mg; Carbohydrates: 2g; Fiber: 1g; Protein: 51g; Iron: 3mg*

Chicken Puttanesca

» Low-Carb

» Serves 2

» Prep time: 20 minutes
Cook time: 20 minutes

Puttanesca is the perfect last-minute, throw-it-together meal because it uses mostly pantry ingredients. In this recipe, we serve the chicken with Toasted Fennel Spaghetti Squash (page 114), but for a lighter dish, you can also serve it over a bed of spinach or other mixed greens.

2 cups Toasted Fennel Spaghetti Squash (page 114), for serving

1 pound cooked boneless, skinless chicken breast, cubed

¼ cup olive oil

2 tablespoons minced garlic

1 tablespoon chopped anchovies (optional)

1 (14½-ounce) can diced tomatoes

1 (14½-ounce) can crushed tomatoes

½ cup kalamata olives, pitted

½ cup quartered artichoke hearts

¼ cup capers

1 teaspoon red pepper flakes

1 teaspoon sea salt

2 tablespoons chopped fresh basil leaves

1. Prepare the spaghetti squash and the chicken breast, if necessary (see the Make It Easier tip after the recipe).

2. Heat the olive oil in a large sauté pan over medium heat. Add the garlic and anchovies (if using) and cook for 1 minute, until fragrant. Add the diced tomatoes, crushed tomatoes, olives, artichokes, capers, red pepper flakes, and salt. Bring the mixture to a boil, stirring occasionally, 5 to 7 minutes.

3. Once the mixture is boiling, reduce the heat to low, add the cooked chicken, and simmer for 15 minutes. Remove from the heat.

4. Serve the chicken puttanesca over the spaghetti squash, garnished with basil.

Make It Easier: To save time, buy precooked chicken breast or cook the chicken breast the night before. To cook the chicken, roast it in the oven at 350°F for 30 minutes, or until its internal temperature reaches 165°F. Cool for 10 minutes, then cut it into cubes to use in this dish.

PER SERVING: *Calories: 753; Total fat: 40g; Sodium: 2943mg; Carbohydrates: 46g; Fiber: 17g; Protein: 58g; Iron: 7mg*

Teriyaki Burgers

» 30 Minutes   » Serves 4   » Prep time: 10 minutes
                                 Cook time: 20 minutes

Burgers are a summertime favorite across the country, and this bun-free recipe uses teriyaki sauce as a sweet and tangy accompaniment to burgers topped with pineapple. This recipe provides instructions for cooking the burgers in a sauté pan, but you can also use a grill. Try serving these over a bed of mixed greens.

For the teriyaki sauce

1 cup coconut aminos
1 cup white wine vinegar
½ cup coconut sugar
1½ teaspoons sea salt

For the burgers

2 pounds ground beef,
    divided and shaped into
    4 burger patties
1½ teaspoons sea salt
½ teaspoon freshly ground
    black pepper
½ tablespoon sesame oil
4 pineapple rings
2 tablespoons olive oil
1 cup shredded cabbage
¼ cup chopped scallions

1. **Make the teriyaki sauce.** In a small saucepan over medium-high heat, combine the coconut aminos, white wine vinegar, coconut sugar, and salt and bring to a boil. Reduce the heat to low and simmer until thickened, about 20 minutes. Remove from the heat and set aside.

2. **Make the burgers.** Season the burger patties with salt and pepper and set aside.

3. Heat the sesame oil in a large sauté pan over medium-high heat. Once hot, add the pineapple rings to the pan and cook for 1 minute on each side, until slightly charred. Remove the pineapple from the pan and set aside.

4. In the same sauté pan, add the olive oil and heat for 1 minute. Once heated, add the patties to the pan and cook for 5 to 7 minutes on each side, depending on your preferred temperature. Remove from the heat and let the burgers rest for 5 minutes.

5. To serve, spoon the teriyaki sauce over each burger. Top with grilled pineapple, shredded cabbage, and scallions and serve immediately. Refrigerate extra teriyaki sauce in an airtight container for up to 2 weeks.

PER SERVING: *Calories: 482; Total fat: 20g; Sodium: 1976mg; Carbohydrates: 23g; Fiber: 1g; Protein: 52g; Iron: 6mg*

Tilapia Fish Tacos

» 30 Minutes, Low-Carb, Diabetes-Friendly

» Serves 2

» Prep time: 10 minutes
Cook time: 15 minutes

California-style fish tacos are often made with fried or grilled fish and topped with a creamy sauce and cabbage. Our healthy version pairs marinated, seasoned tilapia with Creamy Kale Slaw (page 50) and we serve them in lettuce cups. You can also serve these tacos with Paleo-friendly tortillas—our favorite brand is Siete.

For the tilapia

Zest and juice of 1 lime
4 tablespoons olive oil, divided
1 pound tilapia fillets
2 teaspoons chili powder
1 teaspoon paprika
2 teaspoons sea salt
1 teaspoon freshly ground black pepper
½ teaspoon ground cumin
½ teaspoon cayenne pepper

For serving

1 cup Creamy Kale Slaw (page 50)
4 large romaine lettuce leaves
1 small jalapeño, cut into thin rounds
1 avocado, diced
¼ cup chopped cilantro
2 lime wedges, for serving

1. Prepare the slaw.

2. In a shallow dish, combine the lime zest and juice with 1 tablespoon olive oil. Place the tilapia in the oil mixture and marinate for 10 minutes, flipping halfway through.

3. **Make the seasoning blend.** In a small mixing bowl, combine the chili powder, paprika, salt, pepper, cumin, and cayenne pepper and mix to blend. Remove the fish from the marinade and season both sides with the seasoning.

4. Heat the remaining 3 tablespoons olive oil in a non-stick sauté pan over medium-high heat. Carefully add the fish to the pan and cook for 3 to 5 minutes per side, until it is opaque and flakes easily when pierced with a fork. Rest the fish for 5 minutes before gently tearing it into bite-size pieces.

5. To serve, portion the tilapia into the romaine leaves. Top with Creamy Kale Slaw, jalapeño, avocado, and cilantro. Serve with lime wedges on the side.

Ingredient Swaps: Try preparing these tacos with fried tilapia. Use the instructions in the Shrimp Po'Boy recipe (page 90) to create the dredging mixture and fry the dredged tilapia on each side for 3 to 5 minutes.

PER SERVING: *Calories: 807; Total fat: 60g; Sodium: 1537mg; Carbohydrates: 25g; Fiber: 12g; Protein: 51g; Iron: 4mg*

Toasted Fennel Spaghetti Squash

» One-Pot, Vegetarian, Low-Carb, Diabetes-Friendly

» Serves 2

» Prep time: 5 minutes
Cook time: 30 minutes

Spaghetti squash makes a great Paleo-friendly substitute for pasta, because when it's cooked, its flesh falls from the skin in strings, almost like noodles. Slightly sweet in flavor, spaghetti squash pairs nicely with the warm notes of fennel seed and black pepper. When preparing the spaghetti squash, try saving the seeds and toasting them with olive oil and salt. Use the toasted seeds as a salad topping or eat them plain as a snack.

1 large or 2 small
　spaghetti squash
2 cups vegetable stock
2 teaspoons sea salt
½ teaspoon freshly ground
　black pepper
1 tablespoon ground
　toasted fennel seeds
¼ teaspoon red pepper
　flakes, for garnish
¼ cup chopped fresh
　parsley, for garnish
1 tablespoon nutritional
　yeast, for garnish
1 tablespoon fresh
　chopped basil leaves,
　for garnish

1. Preheat the oven to 400°F.

2. Cut the spaghetti squash in half lengthwise and use a spoon to scoop out the seeds. Discard the seeds or reserve for use in another recipe.

3. Place the squash in a casserole dish, cut-side down. Add the stock to the dish and tightly wrap it with aluminum foil. Bake the squash for 30 minutes, or until a knife can easily pierce its skin.

4. Remove the dish from the oven and allow to cool for 15 minutes, or until the squash can be handled. Using a fork, gently rake out the flesh of the squash in spaghetti-like strands into a medium bowl. Toss with the salt, black pepper, and fennel seeds.

5. Divide the squash onto two plates and garnish with red pepper flakes, parsley, nutritional yeast, and basil.

Make It Easier: To cut down on prep work, cook the spaghetti squash in a slow cooker. Halve and deseed the squash prior to cooking; then, for a medium squash, cook it on the low setting for 6 hours.

PER SERVING: *Calories: 103; Total fat: 2g; Sodium: 1542mg; Carbohydrates: 22g; Fiber: 5g; Protein: 2g; Iron: 2mg*

Mushroom Bolognese

» One-Pot, Vegetarian, Low-Carb, Diabetes-Friendly

» Serves 2

» Prep time: 10 minutes
Cook time: 25 minutes

Bolognese is a meat-based sauce made with celery, carrots, beef, and fatty pork, with milk or cream stirred in just before serving. We've adjusted this classic dish to make it both vegetarian and Paleo-compliant. Instead of pork or beef, we use mushrooms, which provide the same rich umami flavor.

¼ cup olive oil

1 small onion, finely chopped

1 medium carrot, finely chopped

1 celery stalk, finely chopped

1 pound button and/or shiitake mushrooms, coarsely chopped

¼ cup tomato paste

2 (14½-ounce) cans crushed tomatoes

1 tablespoon minced garlic

1 tablespoon chopped fresh basil

1 tablespoon chopped fresh sage

2 teaspoons sea salt

1 teaspoon freshly ground black pepper

⅛ teaspoon red pepper flakes

¼ cup full-fat coconut milk

1. Heat the olive oil in a large pot over medium heat. Once the oil is hot, add the onion, carrots, celery, and mushrooms and cook, stirring occasionally, until tender, about 10 minutes.

2. Add the tomato paste to the pot, stir to incorporate, and cook for 2 to 3 minutes, until it begins to brown. Add the crushed tomatoes, garlic, basil, sage, salt, black pepper, and red pepper flakes. Reduce the heat to a simmer and continue to cook for 15 minutes. Remove from the heat, stir in the coconut milk, and serve hot.

Ingredient Swaps: This recipe calls for button and shiitake mushrooms, but you can use any mushrooms in this dish—try using portabella or oyster mushrooms for an earthier flavor.

PER SERVING: *Calories: 504; Total fat: 36g; Sodium: 1287mg; Carbohydrates: 45g; Fiber: 17g; Protein: 12g; Iron: 6mg*

Portabella Fajitas

» Vegetarian, Low-Carb, Diabetes-Friendly

» Serves 2

» Prep time: 10 minutes
Cook time: 25 minutes

Fajitas are a crowd-pleasing dish, and this hands-off sheet pan version makes preparation a breeze: Simply toss the vegetables with spices and bake until crispy. If serving the fajitas on tortillas, we recommend the brand Siete, found online or at health food stores. Try topping these fajitas with sliced avocado or with Bacon-Jalapeño Guacamole (page 52).

2 tablespoons olive oil, divided

2 teaspoons chili powder

½ teaspoon ground cumin

½ teaspoon smoked paprika

2 teaspoons garlic powder

1 teaspoon sea salt

1 teaspoon freshly ground black pepper

1 pound portabella mushrooms, cleaned and cut into ½-inch strips

3 bell peppers, cut into ½-inch strips

1 red onion, cut into ½-inch strips

1 jalapeño, thinly sliced

1 bunch cilantro, chopped

Zest and juice of 1 lime

4 (6- to 8-inch) Paleo-compliant tortillas, for serving (optional)

1. Preheat the oven to 425°F. Lightly coat a baking sheet with 1 tablespoon olive oil.

2. **Make the seasoning mix.** In a small bowl, combine the chili powder, cumin, paprika, garlic powder, salt, and pepper.

3. In a large bowl, combine the mushrooms, bell peppers, onion, and jalapeño. Add the remaining 1 tablespoon olive oil and the seasoning mix and toss to coat.

4. Lay the vegetables in a single layer on the baking sheet and roast for 25 minutes, or until the vegetables are crispy and have begun to char.

5. Remove the fajita vegetables from the oven and stir in the cilantro and lime zest and juice. Serve the fajitas immediately, on their own or with Paleo-friendly tortillas (if using).

Ingredient Swaps: Try preparing these fajitas with bite-size pieces of chicken, steak, or shrimp instead of or in addition to the portabella mushrooms. If using chicken, make sure that its internal temperature reaches 165°F.

PER SERVING: *Calories: 296; Total fat: 16g; Sodium: 692mg; Carbohydrates: 38g; Fiber: 8g; Protein: 9g; Iron: 3mg*

Honey-Jalapeño Seared Pork Tenderloin

» Serves 2

» Prep time: 5 minutes
Cook time: 30 minutes,
plus 10 minutes resting

Pork tenderloin, sometimes called pork filet or gentleman's cut, is the most tender cut of meat in a pig. In this recipe, we pair this tender cut of pork with a slightly sweet, slightly spicy sauce. The sweet coconut aminos in the sauce are balanced with apple cider vinegar for a bit of tanginess. To reduce the spiciness, use only half of a jalapeño.

1 teaspoon sesame oil

½ tablespoon
minced garlic

1 tablespoon coconut
aminos

1 tablespoon apple
cider vinegar

½ cup honey

1 jalapeño, finely chopped

1 pound pork tender-
loin, cleaned

2 teaspoons sea salt

1 teaspoon freshly ground
black pepper

1. Preheat the oven to 425°F.

2. In a small saucepan over low heat, combine the sesame oil and minced garlic. Cook for 2 to 3 minutes, until warm and fragrant. Add the coconut aminos, apple cider vinegar, and honey and simmer for 5 minutes, stirring occasionally, until the sauce reduces slightly. Remove the pan from the heat and stir in the jalapeño. Set aside.

3. Place the pork on a wire rack in a roasting dish (such as a broiling tray) to allow the fat to drip off during cooking. Rub the pork with salt and pepper. Cover the roasting dish loosely with aluminum foil and roast for 20 to 25 minutes, until the juices run clear and the internal temperature of the pork reaches at least 145°F.

4. Remove the pork from the oven and let rest for 10 minutes, then transfer to a cutting board. Cut into 1-inch pieces at a 45-degree angle. Serve hot, drizzled with the sauce.

Ingredient Swaps: Try using ¼ cup maple syrup in place of the honey in this recipe for an earthier flavor.

PER SERVING: *Calories: 560; Total fat: 10g; Sodium: 1478mg; Carbohydrates: 71g; Fiber: 0g; Protein: 48g; Iron: 3mg*

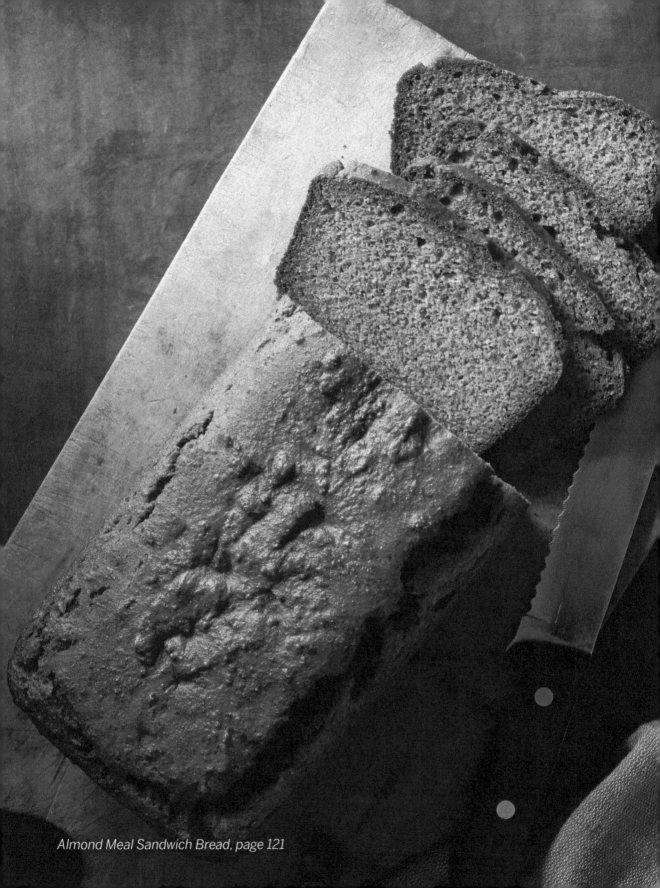

Almond Meal Sandwich Bread, page 121

CHAPTER EIGHT

Breads and Baked Goods

To many, eating bread on the Paleo diet sounds like a contradiction—and for many years, that was true. Thankfully, in recent years, new recipes for Paleo-friendly breads have emerged and become relatively widespread. The star recipe of this chapter is the Almond Meal Sandwich Bread (page 121), which is used in countless recipes throughout this book. We recommend always keeping a loaf on hand. This chapter also includes Paleo takes on many other breads, like Jalapeño-Honey "Corn Bread" (page 122), Tapioca Rolls (page 130), Chocolate Banana Bread (page 123) and even Tortilla Chips (page 125). You'll notice that many Paleo-friendly breads have a different texture and a soft crumb, since they lack the gluten structure of traditional bread, but you can still use them how you would regular bread.

Almond Meal Sandwich Bread

» Low-Carb

» Makes 1
(8-by-4-inch) loaf

» Prep time: 10 minutes
Cook time: 45 minutes

This Paleo-friendly sandwich bread is the foundation of many of the recipes in this book. Made with almond meal, it is naturally high in protein and healthy fats and low in carbohydrates. It is rich, dense, and has a subtle hint of sweetness. This recipe does not use yeast—instead, we rely on the reaction between baking soda and vinegar to produce a slight rise.

Olive oil cooking spray, for greasing the pan
3 cups almond meal
6 tablespoons pumpkin meal
¼ cup coconut flour
½ teaspoon sea salt
1 tablespoon baking soda
9 large eggs
6 tablespoons olive oil
2 tablespoons honey
1 tablespoon plus 2 teaspoons apple cider vinegar

1. Preheat the oven to 350°F and lightly coat an 8-by-4-inch bread loaf pan with olive oil cooking spray.

2. In a medium bowl, combine the almond meal, pumpkin meal, coconut flour, salt, and baking soda and set aside.

3. In the bowl of a stand mixer fitted with the paddle attachment, combine the eggs, olive oil, and honey. Mix on low speed for 2 minutes.

4. While still mixing, use a spatula to slowly add the dry ingredients into the wet ingredients. Continue mixing on low speed for 3 minutes, until fully combined, stopping to scrape down the sides and bottom of the bowl as necessary. Turn off the mixer and use a spatula to gently fold in the apple cider vinegar.

5. Transfer the batter to the loaf pan and bake for 45 minutes. Remove from the oven and allow to cool for at least 20 minutes before serving.

6. Cut into slices or store the loaf whole in a resealable freezer-safe bag. Keep refrigerated for up to 5 days or freeze for up to 6 weeks.

PER SERVING: *Calories: 420; Total fat: 35g; Sodium: 633mg; Carbohydrates: 14g; Fiber: 5g; Protein: 16g; Iron: 3mg*

Jalapeño-Honey "Corn Bread"

» Vegetarian

» Serves 4

» Prep time: 20 minutes
Cook time: 35 to
40 minutes

Corn bread can be sweet or savory, varying by region. Sweet corn bread, common in the northern United States, is soft and almost cake-like in texture, while savory corn bread, common in the South, is firm with a crisp top. This Paleo-friendly "corn bread" uses coconut flour instead of cornmeal and combines some sweet and some savory elements, including honey, applesauce, and jalapeño. Pair it with a BBQ Pulled Pork Sandwich (page 92).

Olive oil cooking spray, for greasing the pan

1 cup coconut flour

1 tablespoon plus
1 teaspoon corn-free baking powder

1 teaspoon sea salt

8 large eggs

1 tablespoon plus
1 teaspoon apple cider vinegar

¼ cup unsweetened applesauce

¼ cup plus
2 tablespoons honey

1 cup olive oil

1 large jalapeño, deseeded and finely diced

1. Preheat the oven to 325°F and lightly coat a 9-by-9-inch baking pan with olive oil cooking spray.

2. In a small bowl, combine the coconut flour, baking powder, and salt and set aside.

3. In the bowl of a stand mixer fitted with the paddle attachment, combine the eggs, apple cider vinegar, applesauce, honey, and olive oil. Mix on low speed until fully incorporated. The mixture will turn a golden-brown color.

4. Continue mixing on low speed and slowly add the dry ingredients. Mix for 5 minutes, stopping as necessary to scrape down the sides and bottom of the bowl. Turn off the mixer and fold the jalapeño into the batter with a spatula.

5. Transfer the batter to the baking pan and bake for 35 minutes, or until set in the center and golden brown on top. Serve hot and refrigerate leftovers in an airtight container for up to 4 days.

PER SERVING: *Calories: 928; Total fat: 67g; Sodium: 460mg; Carbohydrates: 41g; Fiber: 10g; Protein: 19g; Iron: 5mg*

Chocolate Banana Bread

» Vegetarian » Serves 3 » Prep time: 10 minutes
Cook time: 50 minutes

This recipe is great for using up overripe bananas—we peel and freeze all our overripe bananas to save for baking. This Chocolate Banana Bread makes a great breakfast on the go. For a decadent dessert, melt 1 tablespoon coconut oil in a sauté pan, add the banana bread, and sear over medium heat for 4 minutes on each side, until it begins to brown. Enjoy with Vanilla Bean Ice Cream (page 135).

Olive oil cooking spray, for greasing the pan

3 ripe bananas

¼ cup olive oil

2 large eggs

1 tablespoon vanilla extract

1¼ cups almond meal

¼ cup tapioca starch

¼ cup arrowroot starch

2 tablespoons flax meal

1 teaspoon cinnamon

1 teaspoon baking soda

1 teaspoon corn-free baking powder

½ teaspoon sea salt

½ cup walnuts

¼ cup Paleo-friendly chocolate chips, such as Santa Barbara Chocolate's chocolate chips

1. Preheat the oven to 350°F and lightly coat an 8½-by-4½-inch loaf pan with olive oil cooking spray.

2. Add the bananas to the bowl of a stand mixer fitted with the paddle attachment and mix on low speed for 1 minute. Add the olive oil, eggs, and vanilla and continue mixing on low speed for 2 minutes.

3. In a small mixing bowl, combine the almond meal, tapioca starch, arrowroot starch, flax meal, cinnamon, baking soda, baking powder, and sea salt.

4. With the mixer still on low speed, slowly add the dry ingredients. Mix for 3 minutes, stopping as necessary to scrape down the sides of the bowl with a spatula. Turn off the mixer and gently fold in the walnuts and chocolate chips.

5. Transfer the batter to the loaf pan and bake for 50 minutes, rotating the pan halfway through to ensure even browning. Allow to cool for at least 10 minutes; then slice and serve warm. Refrigerate the banana bread wrapped in plastic wrap for up to 1 week or freeze for up to 2 months.

PER SERVING: *Calories: 846; Total fat: 60g; Sodium: 669mg; Carbohydrates: 65g; Fiber: 13g; Protein: 19g; Iron: 5mg*

Chocolate and Pistachio Biscotti

» Vegetarian » Serves 2 » Prep time: 15 minutes
Cook time: 55 minutes

Biscotti comes from the Latin word *biscotus*, which means "twice-cooked" and refers to the way biscotti is prepared. Biscotti are dry biscuits, baked twice to remove all moisture so they can be stored for long periods of time. Try this biscotti dipped in coffee—the toasty flavors pair perfectly with the rich chocolate and floral pistachio.

2 cups almond meal
¼ cup coconut flour
½ cup cocoa powder
1 teaspoon baking soda
½ teaspoon sea salt
½ cup honey
½ cup olive oil
½ cup unsalted pistachios, shelled
¼ cup Paleo-friendly chocolate chips, such as Santa Barbara Chocolate's chocolate chips

1. Preheat the oven to 325°F and line a 9-by-9-inch baking pan with parchment paper.

2. In a medium mixing bowl, combine the almond meal, coconut flour, cocoa powder, baking soda, and salt.

3. In the bowl of a stand mixer fitted with the paddle attachment, combine the honey and olive oil. While mixing on low speed, slowly add the dry ingredients. Continue mixing for 2 minutes, until a dough forms. Fold in the pistachios and chocolate chips.

4. Transfer the dough to the baking pan and use your hands to shape it into a mound, roughly 6 inches long and 4 inches wide.

5. Bake the dough for 30 minutes, then remove the pan from the oven and place it in the refrigerator to chill for 30 minutes.

6. Preheat the oven again to 325°F. Line a baking sheet with parchment paper for the second bake.

7. Once cooled, use a sharp knife to cut the biscotti into six 1-inch-thick slices. Lay the slices flat on the baking sheet. Bake for an additional 15 minutes. Serve or store biscotti in an airtight container for up to 2 weeks.

PER SERVING: *Calories: 1671; Total fat: 127g; Sodium: 945mg; Carbohydrates: 129g; Fiber: 28g; Protein: 35g; Iron: 12mg*

Tortilla Chips

Corn tortilla chips are not permitted on the Paleo diet, but with this healthy and delicious oven-baked recipe you can enjoy homemade chips. The almond flour used in these gives them an almost sweet flavor. For this recipe, it is important to use blanched almond flour for its lighter texture. Serve with Bacon-Jalapeño Guacamole (page 52) or Baba Ghanoush (page 53).

2½ cups almond flour or
blanched almond meal
1½ teaspoons chia seeds
or flaxseed
1 teaspoon sea salt
2 large eggs
1½ teaspoons freshly
squeezed lemon juice

1. Preheat the oven to 325°F.

2. In a large mixing bowl, combine the almond flour, chia seeds, and salt and stir to combine. Use a spoon to make a small well in the center of the mixture. Pour the eggs and lemon juice into the well and stir until a dough starts to form. Use your hands to finish mixing, pulling the dough into a ball.

3. Lay an 18-inch sheet of parchment paper on the kitchen counter. Place the ball of dough in the center and top with another 18-inch sheet of parchment paper. Use your palm to flatten the dough slightly. Then, using a rolling pin, start from the center of the dough and begin rolling it outward. Continue working from the center to roll the dough as thin as possible—it should reach the edges of the parchment paper.

4. Remove the top layer of parchment paper and use a pizza cutter to score the dough in a grid, making 2-inch squares. Carefully transfer the parchment paper directly onto the oven rack and bake for 16 to 20 minutes, until golden brown. Serve hot and store extra chips in an airtight container for up to 3 days.

PER SERVING: *Calories: 777; Total fat: 65g; Sodium: 654mg; Carbohydrates: 28g; Fiber: 16g; Protein: 32g; Iron: 6mg*

Nut and Seed Granola

» 30 Minutes

» Serves 2

» Prep time: 5 minutes
Cook time: 20 minutes

Not many people know that granola was developed in the late 1800s by a health-care reformer. Although originally intended to be a health food, many commercial granolas available today are loaded with added sugars and include grains, which are not Paleo-compliant. Our simple, healthy granola combines nuts and seeds with a touch of honey and chocolate.

½ cup slivered almonds

½ cup pumpkin seeds

2 tablespoons
  Paleo-friendly chocolate
  chips, such as Santa
  Barbara Chocolate's
  chocolate chips

1 tablespoon chia seeds

1 tablespoon cocoa powder

¼ cup sunflower seeds

1 tablespoon
  almond butter

1 tablespoon honey

¼ teaspoon sea salt

½ teaspoon vanilla extract

¼ teaspoon nutmeg

1. Preheat the oven to 300°F and line a baking sheet with parchment paper.

2. In a small bowl, combine the almonds, pumpkin seeds, chocolate chips, chia seeds, cocoa powder, sunflower seeds, almond butter, honey, salt, vanilla, and nutmeg. Stir with a spatula until thoroughly combined.

3. Transfer the mixture to the baking sheet and spread it out in a single layer. Bake for 20 minutes, until golden brown. Cool for 10 minutes before serving. Store leftover granola in an airtight container for up to 3 weeks.

Ingredient Swaps: Try replacing the chocolate chips and cocoa powder in this recipe with any unsweetened dried fruit of your choice.

PER SERVING: *Calories: 584; Total fat: 46g; Sodium: 166mg; Carbohydrates: 31g; Fiber: 12g; Protein: 22g; Iron: 6mg*

Garlic-Herb Croutons or Bread Crumbs

» 5-Ingredient, 30 Minutes, Low-Carb, Diabetes-Friendly

» Makes 1½ cups

» Prep time: 5 minutes
Cook time: 20 minutes

This recipe uses Almond Meal Sandwich Bread as its base, so these croutons are high in protein and low in carbohydrates. We incorporate lemon zest and juice, which give the croutons a touch of brightness and help preserve freshness over time. Serve these croutons over the top of Classic Wedge Salad with "Bleu Cheese" Dressing (page 71) or Curried Tomato Soup (page 88) or crush them to make bread crumbs for use with several recipes in this book.

3 slices Almond Meal Sandwich Bread (page 121), cut into ¾-inch cubes.

¼ teaspoon minced garlic

¼ teaspoon Italian seasoning

Zest and juice of ½ lemon

⅛ teaspoon sea salt

1. Prepare the bread, if necessary.

2. Preheat the oven to 300°F and line a baking sheet with parchment paper.

3. In a small mixing bowl, combine the bread cubes with the garlic, Italian seasoning, lemon zest and juice, and salt. Toss to evenly coat.

4. Spread the seasoned croutons on the baking sheet and bake for 20 minutes, flipping halfway through, until the croutons are hard. Serve immediately or refrigerate in an airtight container for up to 1 week.

5. To make Paleo-friendly bread crumbs, place the croutons to the bowl of a food processor. Pulse for 30 seconds, or until the croutons crumble into a fine powder. Keep the bread crumbs refrigerated in an airtight container for up to 2 weeks, or frozen for up to 2 months.

Scale It Up: As long as they're baked all of the way through and don't come into contact with moisture, these croutons will stay fresh for up to 1 week. Double or triple this recipe to enjoy in salads all week long.

PER SERVING: *Calories: 315; Total fat: 26g; Sodium: 475mg; Carbohydrates: 10g; Fiber: 3g; Protein: 12g; Iron: 2mg*

Pizza Crust

» 30 Minutes,
  5-Ingredient

» Serves 2

» Prep time: 5 minutes
  Cook time: 25 minutes

One of the first versions of the dish we now know as pizza was served in Italy as a flatbread with simple toppings: soft mozzarella, fresh tomatoes, and basil. This style, called margherita pizza, is still popular today. To make Paleo-friendly flatbread-style pizza, bake this crust topped with tomato sauce or Nut-Free Pesto (page 157) and vegetables (like mushrooms, olives, and spinach).

Olive oil cooking spray, for
  greasing the pan
2½ cups tapioca starch
½ teaspoon sea salt
1 teaspoon Italian
  seasoning
½ cup olive oil
½ cup water
2 large eggs, beaten

1. Preheat the oven to 300°F and lightly coat a baking sheet with olive oil cooking spray.

2. In a medium bowl, combine the tapioca starch, salt, and Italian seasoning and stir to combine.

3. Combine the olive oil and water in a small microwave-safe bowl and microwave on high power for 1 minute.

4. Transfer the oil mixture to the bowl of a stand mixer fitted with the paddle attachment. Add the eggs and mix on low speed for 1 minute. While mixing, slowly add the dry mixture to the wet mixture. Continue mixing on low speed for 2 minutes.

5. Transfer the pizza dough to the baking sheet and use a spatula to spread it as thin as possible, making sure not to leave any gaps. If your spatula is sticking to the dough, coat it with cooking spray.

6. Bake the dough for 20 to 25 minutes, or until slightly brown on the edges.

7. If serving immediately, top with toppings of your choice and enjoy hot. Or, freeze the crust for later use by wrapping it tightly in plastic wrap and then placing it in a freezer-safe resealable bag. Store frozen for up to 8 weeks. To use, thaw it to room temperature.

Scale It Up: Since this recipe keeps well in the freezer, double it to have one crust for now and one crust for later.

PER SERVING: *Calories: 1217; Total fat: 59g; Sodium: 363mg; Carbohydrates: 162g; Fiber: 0g; Protein: 6g; Iron: 1mg*

Tapioca Rolls

» 5-Ingredient,
   30 Minutes

» Serves 2

» Prep time: 5 minutes
   Cook time: 20 minutes

Dinner rolls make a great side for any meal and are also a great option for small sandwiches or sliders. Many dinner rolls are made with wheat flour and sugar, but we use tapioca starch instead—a preparation also used in Korean and Brazilian cooking. Tapioca flour has a neutral flavor and thickens at lower temperatures, creating structure and chewiness in the bread without any rising time.

Olive oil cooking spray, for greasing the pan

1 cup tapioca starch

¼ teaspoon sea salt

2 teaspoons coconut flour

½ teaspoon nutritional yeast

6 tablespoons water

4 tablespoons olive oil

1 large egg, beaten

1. Preheat the oven to 350°F and lightly coat a baking sheet with olive oil cooking spray.

2. In a medium bowl, combine the tapioca starch, salt, coconut flour, and nutritional yeast. Stir to incorporate.

3. Combine the water and olive oil in a small microwave-safe bowl. Microwave on high power for 1 minute.

4. Pour the liquid mixture into the flour mixture and begin stirring. A gel will begin to form. Add the egg and continue mixing vigorously with a whisk, until all the ingredients are well incorporated.

5. Use a ¼-cup measuring cup to drop the dough directly onto the baking sheet, spaced a few inches apart—the dough should yield 4 rolls.

6. Bake the rolls for 30 minutes, then let them rest for at least 10 minutes before serving.

Ingredient Swaps: This dough is a great, neutral base recipe. Try adding your favorite herbs and seasonings for different flavor profiles. We love adding fresh garlic and Italian seasoning or olives and rosemary.

PER SERVING: *Calories: 494; Total fat: 29g; Sodium: 191mg; Carbohydrates: 52g; Fiber: 0g; Protein: 3g; Iron: 1mg*

Bread Crumb Dressing

» 30 Minutes, Low-Carb, Diabetes-Friendly

» Serves 4

» Prep time: 10 minutes
Cook time: 20 minutes

The ingredients for dressing and stuffing—both traditional holiday favorites—are technically the same, but the method of preparation is different. Stuffing is cooked inside of a turkey, while dressing is baked separately in a dish. Our festive Paleo-compliant stuffing is made with high-protein, low-carb Garlic-Herb Croutons (page 127) in place of wheat bread.

2 tablespoons olive oil

½ small yellow onion, diced

2 stalks celery, diced

1 tablespoon dried parsley

3 cups Garlic-Herb Croutons (page 127)

2 large eggs, hard-boiled and diced

1½ cups chicken stock

1 teaspoon sea salt

½ teaspoon freshly ground black pepper

½ teaspoon ground sage

½ teaspoon dried rosemary

½ teaspoon dried thyme

1. Prepare the croutons, if necessary.

2. Preheat the oven to 350°F.

3. Heat the olive oil in a medium sauté pan over medium heat. Once hot, add the onion, celery, and parsley. Sauté for 4 minutes, stirring frequently, until the onion is soft and translucent. Remove from the heat and set aside.

4. In a medium mixing bowl, combine the croutons, eggs, stock, salt, pepper, sage, rosemary, and thyme.

5. Add the sautéed onions and celery to the crouton mixture and toss to combine. Make sure the croutons soak up the liquid.

6. Transfer the mixture to an 8-by-8-inch baking dish and bake for 20 minutes, or until the center is set. Serve hot.

Ingredient Swaps: Try adding ½ cup fresh cranberries and ¼ cup walnuts to the mix prior to baking for a slightly sweet, slightly tart flavor profile. If adding the fresh fruit, omit the hard-boiled eggs, add ¼ cup stock, and bake for an additional 10 minutes.

PER SERVING: *Calories: 419; Total fat: 35g; Sodium: 805mg; Carbohydrates: 12g; Fiber: 3g; Protein: 15g; Iron: 2mg*

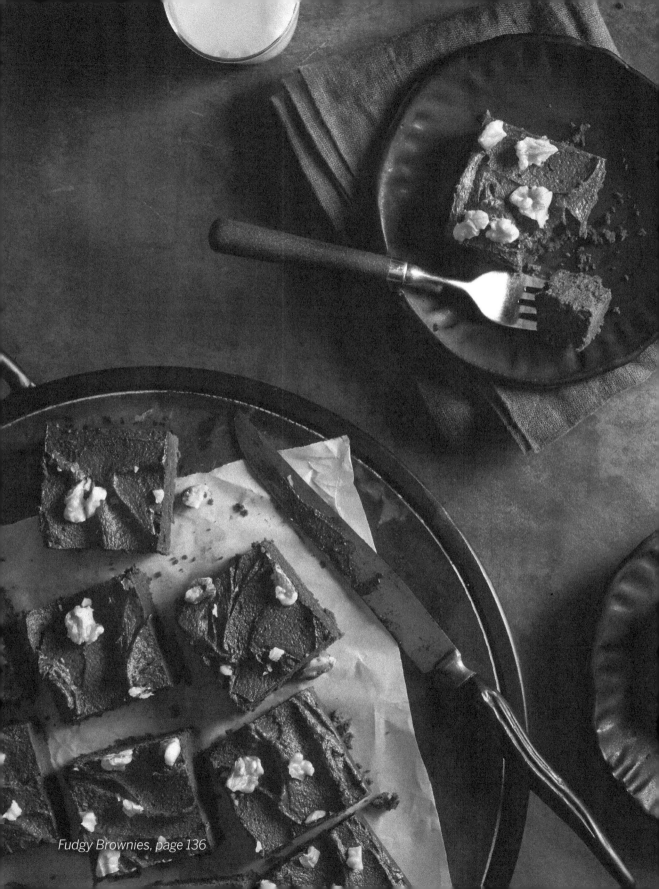

Fudgy Brownies, page 136

CHAPTER NINE

Desserts

— ◇ —

No cookbook—not even a Paleo cookbook—is complete without desserts. To make it easy for you to make a variety of Paleo-compliant and delicious desserts for all occasions, we've come up with 10 recipes designed for those of us with a sweet tooth. Celebrate a birthday with our Chocolate Cake (page 142) iced with Dark Chocolate Frosting (page 147) and served with Vanilla Bean Ice Cream (page 135). Enjoy a Coconut Almond Truffle (page 138) or an Almond Butter Cup (page 144) as an after-dinner treat. Or make Sweet Potato Pie (page 140) or Pecan Pie Bars (page 146), both perfect holiday desserts. Start baking and see all the possibilities for yourself.

Many people mistakenly believe that they won't be able to enjoy chocolate after switching to Paleo, but there are a couple of great options. Unsweetened cocoa powder is Paleo-compliant, and there are also Paleo-friendly chocolate chips available. We recommend Santa Barbara Chocolate's organic chocolate chips, which are sweetened with coconut sugar and made with palm oil rather than soybean oil.

Vanilla Bean Ice Cream

» One-Pot, 5-Ingredient, Vegetarian

» Serves 4

» Prep time: 5 minutes, plus at least 1 hour to freeze
Cook time: 20 to 40 minutes

Ice cream is typically made with cream, sugar, and eggs. For this Paleo-friendly recipe, we replace the cream with coconut milk and the sugar with maple syrup and use tapioca as a binder in place of eggs. This coconut ice cream isn't as rich as dairy ice cream, but it is delicious in its own way—light, airy, and sure to satisfy your sweet tooth.

2 (13½-ounce) cans full-fat coconut milk, chilled
½ tablespoon vanilla extract
⅓ cup maple syrup
¼ teaspoon kosher salt
1 teaspoon tapioca starch

1. Freeze the bowl of your ice cream maker ahead of time, according to the manufacturer's instructions.

2. In a blender, combine the coconut milk, vanilla, maple syrup, salt, and tapioca starch. Blend on high speed for 1 minute, or until smooth and fully incorporated.

3. Place the prefrozen bowl into the ice cream maker. Pour the mixture into the bowl, turn the machine on, and churn according to the manufacturer's instructions, usually between 20 and 40 minutes.

4. Once the ice cream is finished churning, serve immediately or, for firmer ice cream, freeze in an airtight container for at least one hour. Keep leftovers frozen for up to 1 week.

Ingredient Swaps: For firmer ice cream, replace the tapioca starch with ground psyllium husk, a powder made from the seeds of the *Plantago ovata* plant that is available at most health food stores. Use 4 teaspoons psyllium husk for every 1 teaspoon tapioca starch.

PER SERVING: *Calories: 466; Total fat: 42g; Sodium: 107mg; Carbohydrates: 24g; Fiber: 0g; Protein: 4g; Iron: 7mg*

Fudgy Brownies

» Vegetarian   » Makes 9 brownies   » Prep time: 10 minutes
Cook time: 35 minutes

These decadent Fudgy Brownies make use of two Paleo-friendly sweeteners—honey and coconut sugar—as well as instant coffee, which brings out the varied flavors of the chocolate. Be sure to whip the eggs for a full 3 minutes until fluffy, as this will help the brownies retain their structure.

Olive oil cooking spray, for greasing the pan
3 large eggs
1 cup coconut sugar
2 cups almond meal
2 tablespoons coconut flour
2 tablespoons cocoa powder
1 tablespoon instant coffee
1 cup Paleo-friendly chocolate chips, such as Santa Barbara Chocolate's chocolate chips
½ cup plus 2 tablespoons olive oil

1. Preheat the oven to 300°F and lightly coat a 9-by-9-inch baking pan with olive oil spray.

2. In the bowl of a stand mixer fitted with the whisk attachment, combine the eggs and coconut sugar. Whisk on medium-high speed for 3 minutes, until light and frothy.

3. In a small mixing bowl, combine the almond meal, coconut flour, cocoa powder, and instant coffee.

4. Adjust a stand mixer to low speed and slowly add the dry ingredients. Mix on medium-low speed for 2 minutes, until fully combined.

5. In a small microwave-safe bowl, combine the chocolate chips and olive oil. Microwave on medium power in 30-second intervals, stirring after each interval, until melted. Turn off the mixer and use a spatula to gently fold the melted chocolate into the batter.

6. Transfer the batter to the pan and bake for 30 to 35 minutes, until a toothpick inserted in the center of the pan comes out clean. Be careful not to overbake the brownies. Cool for 30 minutes at room temperature, then chill for 30 minutes in the refrigerator.

7. Once cooled, use a sharp knife to cut the brownies into nine 3-by-3-inch pieces and serve. Keep brownies refrigerated in an airtight container for up to 5 days, or wrap them individually in plastic wrap and freeze for up to 1 month.

Ingredient Swaps: For an even richer dessert, once cooled, ice the brownies with Dark Chocolate Frosting (page 147) and top with chopped walnuts. Serve with a scoop of Vanilla Bean Ice Cream (page 135).

PER SERVING (1 BROWNIE): *Calories: 458; Total fat: 37g; Sodium: 27mg; Carbohydrates: 29g; Fiber: 1g; Protein: 9g; Iron: 7mg*

Coconut Almond Truffles

» 30 Minutes, Vegetarian   » Makes about 30 truffles   » Prep time: 5 minutes
Cook time: 20 minutes

Bite-size dessert truffles come in many forms. Our recipe uses coconut oil as a base for a creamy filling that is coated in chocolate. Coconut oil works as a filling in this recipe but the melting point is 78°F, so make sure it's cool enough to handle as a solid.

1 cup coconut oil (in a solid state)
2 tablespoons honey
½ teaspoon vanilla extract
1 cup slivered almonds
½ cup unsweetened shredded coconut
2 cups Paleo-friendly chocolate chips, such as Santa Barbara Chocolate's chocolate chips
1 tablespoon cocoa powder

1. In a small bowl, combine the coconut oil, honey, and vanilla. Use a spoon to mix the ingredients together until fully incorporated. Add the almonds and shredded coconut and stir to combine.

2. Line a small baking sheet with parchment paper (it should be able to fit in your freezer). Roll the coconut filling into teaspoon-size balls, about 1 inch in diameter. Space the balls approximately ½ inch apart on the baking sheet. If the filling starts to melt, pause and chill the filling in the refrigerator for 5 to 10 minutes. Once all of the truffles are rolled, put the baking sheet in the freezer for 30 minutes.

3. Place the chocolate chips in a small microwave-safe bowl and microwave on medium power in 30-second increments, stirring after each interval, until fully melted.

4. Remove the coconut oil balls from the freezer. Using two forks, carefully dip the balls into the melted chocolate, allowing any excess chocolate to drip out through the forks. Place the dipped truffle back on the baking sheet and repeat. Once all the truffles are dipped, sprinkle them lightly with the cocoa powder.

5. Keep the truffles frozen in an airtight container for up to 8 weeks.

Ingredient Swaps: Try making these truffles with maple syrup instead of honey for an earthier flavor. Since maple syrup is high in sugar, use just 1 tablespoon.

PER SERVING (2 TRUFFLES): *Calories: 310; Total fat: 32g; Sodium: 4mg; Carbohydrates: 12g; Fiber: 1g; Protein: 3g; Iron: 5mg*

Sweet Potato Pie

» Vegetarian   » Serves 6   » Prep time: 1 hour
                                        Cook time: 1 hour

Sweet potatoes, if stored correctly, can be kept fresh year-round, and you only need two or three sweet potatoes for this delicious pie. This smooth, creamy sweet potato filling is spiced with pumpkin pie spice blend, which contains cinnamon, nutmeg, cloves, all-spice, and ginger. Since sweet potatoes contain natural sugars, this recipe uses very little sugar compared to pumpkin pie, making it a healthy, flavorful alternative.

1 batch Paleo Piecrust
  (page 148), unbaked
2 pounds sweet potatoes,
  scrubbed
6 tablespoons coco-
  nut sugar
3 tablespoons melted
  coconut oil
1 cup full-fat coconut milk
1½ teaspoons pumpkin
  pie spice
1½ teaspoons
  vanilla extract
2 large eggs

1. Preheat the oven to 350°F and line a baking sheet with parchment paper.

2. Make the piecrust, following only steps 1 and 2 of the Paleo Piecrust recipe—you do not need to prebake the crust for this recipe.

3. Place the sweet potatoes whole on the baking sheet and bake for 45 minutes to 1 hour, until the skin can easily be pierced with a fork. Remove them from the oven and set them aside to cool.

4. Once cool enough to handle, use your fingers to peel the skin off of the sweet potatoes. Discard the skin and add the flesh to the bowl of a stand mixer fitted with the paddle attachment. Add the coconut sugar, coconut oil, coconut milk, pumpkin pie spice, vanilla, and eggs. Mix on low speed for 3 to 5 minutes, until creamy in texture.

5. Transfer the batter to the piecrust and bake for 1 hour, until set in the center. Cool for 20 minutes before serving. Keep the pie refrigerated for up to 4 days in an airtight container.

PER SERVING: *Calories: 825; Total fat: 58g; Sodium: 317mg; Carbohydrates: 67g; Fiber: 11g; Protein: 16g; Iron: 5mg*

Pineapple Sorbet

» One-Pot, 5-Ingredient, Low-Carb, Diabetes-Friendly, Vegetarian

» Serves 2

» Prep time: 10 minutes, plus 4 to 7 hours freezing

Sorbet is made by freezing fresh fruit and fruit juice—dairy-free, fat-free, and great for a refreshing Paleo-friendly dessert. This is a great treat to enjoy on a hot summer day for kids and adults alike. Be sure to check the Ingredient Swaps tip after the recipe for ideas on how to switch up the flavors.

1 pineapple, trimmed and core removed

½ cup honey

1 cup water

1 tablespoon lime juice

½ teaspoon sea salt

1 tablespoon finely chopped cilantro leaves (optional)

½ tablespoon minced jalapeño (optional)

1. Cut the pineapple into 1-inch cubes and add it to the bowl of a food processor or a blender. Add the honey, water, lime juice, and salt and blend until pureed, about 2 minutes. Pour the mixture into a freezer-safe container, cover, and freeze it for 1 to 2 hours, until mostly solid.

2. Remove the mixture from the freezer and return it to the food processor or blender. Continue to blend until smooth. Add the cilantro and jalapeño, if using, and pulse a few times to incorporate. Transfer the sorbet back to the freezer-safe container and freeze for 3 to 5 hours before serving. The sorbet will keep in an airtight container for up to 1 week.

Ingredient Swaps: Try this recipe with almost any fruit (or fresh herb)—mango, strawberries, and raspberries all work well. Try different fruit combinations, like peach-mango with mint or a mixed berry blend. Our personal favorite combination is strawberry and basil.

PER SERVING: *Calories: 486; Total fat: 1g; Sodium: 299mg; Carbohydrates: 129g; Fiber: 7g; Protein: 3g; Iron: 2mg*

Chocolate Cake

» Vegetarian

» Makes 1 (2-layer) cake (Serves 8)

» Prep time: 10 minutes
Cook time: 45 minutes, plus 1 hour freezing

Following the Paleo diet doesn't mean you have to miss out on cake. This rich Chocolate Cake pairs perfectly with Dark Chocolate Frosting (page 147). The wet-to-dry ratio in this recipe is greater than you may be accustomed to—this is because coconut flour is very fine and therefore more absorbent than most other flours. This is a supersoft cake, and for that reason, you'll freeze it after baking so it is sturdy enough to release from the cake pans.

Olive oil cooking spray, for greasing the pans
¾ cup coconut flour, sifted
2 teaspoons tapioca starch
½ cup cocoa powder
1 teaspoon sea salt
1 teaspoon baking soda
1 cup olive oil
1¼ cups honey
6 large eggs
1 tablespoon vanilla extract
1 cup Dark Chocolate Frosting (page 147), for icing

1. Preheat the oven to 300°F and lightly coat two 8-inch round cake pans with olive oil cooking spray. Cut a piece of parchment paper to fit in the bottom of each cake pan.

2. In a small mixing bowl, combine the coconut flour, tapioca starch, cocoa powder, sea salt, and baking soda.

3. In the bowl of a stand mixer fitted with the paddle attachment, combine the olive oil, honey, eggs, and vanilla. Mix on low speed for 2 minutes to incorporate. Continue mixing and slowly add the dry ingredients. Mix on low speed for 5 minutes, pausing to scrape down the sides with a spatula as necessary.

4. Divide the batter evenly between the two prepared cake pans and bake for 30 minutes, or until a toothpick inserted in the center of the pan comes out clean. Allow the cake layers to cool for 30 minutes at room temperature. Once cooled, transfer the cake pans to the freezer and freeze for 1 hour.

5. While the cake is freezing, prepare the frosting.

6. Once frozen, remove the cakes from the freezer and run a butter knife around the edge of the pans to release any stuck bits. Flip the cake pans upside down on a cutting board and gently tap the bottoms of the pans to release.

7. If serving immediately, frost the layers. The cake will keep in the refrigerator for up to 5 days. If preparing the cake in advance, wrap the layers separately in plastic wrap and store flat in the freezer for up to 1 month.

Make It Easier: To save on assembly time, make cupcakes instead. Pour this cake batter into a 12-cup muffin tin lined with paper liners. Bake for 25 to 30 minutes, or until a toothpick inserted into a cupcake comes out clean. Cool and frost, if desired.

PER SERVING: *Calories: 711; Total fat: 49g; Sodium: 362mg; Carbohydrates: 66g; Fiber: 7g; Protein: 7g; Iron: 3mg*

Almond Butter Cups

» 5-Ingredient,
Vegetarian

» Makes 6 large cups

» Prep time: 45 minutes

Peanut butter cups are one of our favorite desserts—there's just something irresistible about the combination of chocolate and peanut butter. We knew we had to come up with a Paleo-friendly version. This recipe pairs Paleo-friendly chocolate chips with a creamy almond butter filling. Try chopping them into pieces and serving them on top of Vanilla Bean Ice Cream (page 135).

1 cup Paleo-friendly
   chocolate chips,
   such as Santa
   Barbara Chocolate's
   chocolate chips
½ teaspoon organic palm
   shortening
Olive oil cooking spray, for
   greasing the liners
¼ cup melted coconut oil
½ cup almond butter
¼ cup honey
½ teaspoon sea salt

1. In a small, microwave-safe bowl, combine the chocolate chips and palm shortening. Microwave on medium power in 30-second intervals, stirring after each interval, until fully melted (about 2 minutes total).

2. Line a 6-cup muffin tin with paper liners and lightly coat the liners with olive oil cooking spray. Using a 1-tablespoon measuring spoon, scoop the melted chocolate into each of the six muffin cups. Freeze for 10 minutes, until the chocolate is solid.

3. While the chocolate base freezes, combine the coconut oil, almond butter, honey, and salt in a small mixing bowl and stir to incorporate.

4. Once the chocolate is set, scoop 2 tablespoons of the almond butter filling into each muffin cup, on top of the chocolate. Return the muffin tin to the freezer for 15 minutes, until the filling sets.

5. Remove the muffin tin from the freezer and top each almond butter cup with 1 tablespoon of melted chocolate. Spread to cover the almond butter completely. Return the muffin tin to the freezer for 10 minutes to set.

6. Serve chilled and keep leftovers refrigerated in an airtight container for up to 2 weeks.

Ingredient Swaps: For a crunchier Almond Butter Cup, add 2 tablespoons unsalted chopped almonds to the filling mixture.

PER SERVING (1 CUP): *Calories: 355; Total fat: 31g; Sodium: 99mg; Carbohydrates: 22g; Fiber: 2g; Protein: 6g; Iron: 5mg*

Pecan Pie Bars

» Vegetarian

» Serves 4

» Prep time: 10 minutes
Cook time: 30 minutes,
plus 1 hour to chill

Pecans are the fruit of a hickory tree varietal and appear each year during the fall. Pecans have a high unsaturated fat content, which make them very heart healthy, but this can also cause them to spoil quickly if not handled properly. While this recipe is written as a bar, you can follow the same ingredients and steps to make a Paleo Chocolate Pecan Pie as well.

1 batch Paleo Piecrust
dough (page 148)
Olive oil cooking spray, for
greasing the pan
3 tablespoons honey
3 large eggs
½ teaspoon vanilla extract
1 cup coconut sugar
½ teaspoon sea salt
½ teaspoon cinnamon
⅔ cup Paleo-friendly
chocolate chips, such as
Santa Barbara Choco-
late's chocolate chips
2 cups chopped pecans

1. Make the piecrust dough (step 1 only).

2. Preheat the oven to 300°F and lightly coat an 8-by-8-inch baking pan with olive oil spray.

3. Using your hands, gently press the pie dough into the baking pan in an even layer, making sure it reaches the edges.

4. In the bowl of a stand mixer fitted with the paddle attachment, combine the honey, eggs, and vanilla. Mix on low speed for 1 minute. Add the coconut sugar, salt, cinnamon, chocolate chips, and pecans and continue mixing for 2 minutes.

5. Spread the pecan mixture in an even layer to cover the pie dough. Bake for 30 minutes, then chill for 1 hour in the refrigerator. Using a sharp knife, cut into 9 bars and serve. Refrigerate leftovers in an airtight container for up to 5 days.

Ingredient Swaps: Use maple syrup in place of honey for an even deeper flavor. If you use maple syrup, reduce the amount to 2 tablespoons, since it is sweeter than honey.

PER SERVING: *Calories: 1532; Total fat: 116g; Sodium: 673mg; Carbohydrates: 112g; Fiber: 14g; Protein: 30g; Iron: 10mg*

Dark Chocolate Frosting

» One-Pot, 5-Ingredient, 30 Minutes, Vegetarian

» Makes 2 cups

» Prep time: 10 minutes

This rich and creamy chocolate frosting is the perfect addition to our Chocolate Cake (page 142) and Fudgy Brownies (page 136), but it is also good enough to eat plain with a spoon! Because honey is sticky, it can be difficult to measure—lightly coat your measuring cup with olive oil cooking spray before measuring, and the honey will slide right out.

1¼ cups organic palm oil shortening

⅓ cup arrowroot starch

¼ cup plus 3 tablespoons unsweetened cocoa powder

½ cup honey

½ teaspoon vanilla extract

1. In the bowl of a stand mixer fitted with the paddle attachment, cream the palm oil shortening for 3 minutes.

2. Turn off the mixer and add the arrowroot starch and cocoa powder. Turn the mixer back on at low speed and mix for 3 minutes. Use a spatula to scrape down the sides to ensure the mixture is fully combined.

3. Continue mixing on low speed and pour in the honey and vanilla. Increase the speed to medium and mix until fluffy and whipped, about 3 minutes.

4. Refrigerate the frosting in an airtight container for up to 3 weeks. Remove from the refrigerator 2 hours before using to allow the frosting to return to room temperature.

Ingredient Swaps: You can use the same amount of tapioca starch as a direct substitute for the arrowroot starch—both act as stabilizers in this recipe.

PER SERVING: *Calories: 393; Total fat: 34g; Sodium: 2mg; Carbohydrates: 25g; Fiber: 2g; Protein: 1g; Iron: 1mg*

Paleo Piecrust

» 5-Ingredient, 30
Minutes, Low-Carb,
Diabetes-Friendly,
Vegetarian

» Makes 1 piecrust

» Prep time: 15 minutes
Cook time: 15 minutes
(if prebaking)

Every baker needs a good piecrust recipe. Piecrusts are traditionally made with flour, cold butter, and eggs. Our Paleo recipe uses almond meal in place of flour and palm shortening instead of butter. The almond meal gives this crust a slightly sweet, nutty flavor. Use this crust for Sweet Potato Pie (page 140) or as a base for Pecan Pie Bars (page 146).

2²/₃ cups almond meal
²/₃ cup tapioca starch
1 teaspoon sea salt
2 large eggs
½ cup organic palm oil
shortening
1½ teaspoons
vanilla extract
Olive oil cooking spray, for
greasing the pan

1. In the bowl of a stand mixer fitted with the paddle attachment, combine the almond meal, tapioca starch, and salt. Mix for 30 seconds on low speed. Turn off the mixer and add the eggs, palm oil shortening, and vanilla. Continue mixing on low speed for 2 minutes—the dough should come together to form a ball.

2. Lightly coat a 9-inch pie dish with olive oil cooking spray. Press the dough ball to the center of the pie pan and use the palms of your hands to begin to flatten the dough across the pie dish, pushing out from the center until it reaches the rim. Ensure there are no gaps and that the dough is in an even layer. If the dough becomes sticky, dust your hands with tapioca starch and pat the dough smooth. Keep refrigerated until use, up to 1 week.

3. If you are preparing a no-bake pie, prebake the piecrust for 15 minutes at 300°F and let cool before adding the filling. For a baked pie, add the filling and bake according to the pie's instructions.

Scale It Up: Double this recipe. To freeze, wrap the dough tightly in plastic wrap and keep frozen for 4 to 6 weeks. When ready to use, defrost the dough for 1 hour at room temperature before baking.

PER SERVING: *Calories: 725; Total fat: 61g; Sodium: 327mg; Carbohydrates: 33g; Fiber: 9g; Protein: 17g; Iron: 3mg*

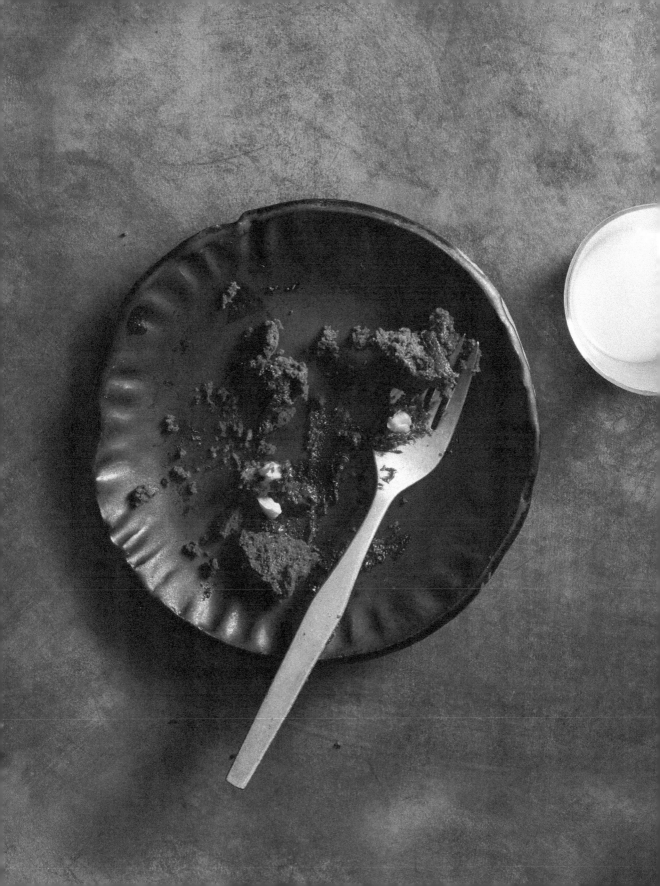

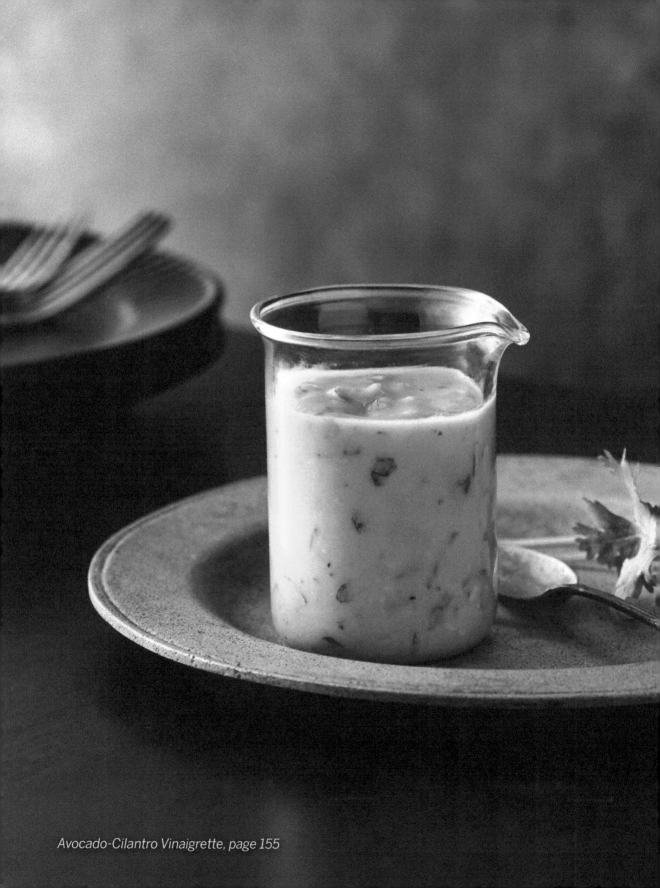

Avocado-Cilantro Vinaigrette, page 155

CHAPTER TEN

Staples, Sauces, and Dressings

— ◇ —

If we had to choose one chapter that is most useful for sticking to the Paleo lifestyle, this would be it. So many store-bought sauces are packed with processed ingredients, so learning how to make homemade versions can take your Paleo cooking to the next level. This chapter provides 11 staple sauces and dressings to elevate otherwise-plain dishes, like grilled chicken or roasted vegetables, into meals you'll enjoy time and time again.

Basics include Paleo Mayo (page 156), Guilt-Free Ranch Dressing (page 160), BBQ Sauce (page 158) and Zesty Ketchup (page 162). Once you master these, move on to Nut-Free Pesto (page 157) to spruce up oven-baked chicken or salmon. The recipes for these sauces and dressings make large batches, and most will keep for a couple of weeks or longer, so you can use make them ahead and use them in several recipes.

Basic Vinaigrette

» One-Pot, 5-Ingredient, 30 Minutes, Low-Carb, Diabetes-Friendly, Vegetarian

» Makes 1 cup

» Prep time: 5 minutes

A vinaigrette is made by combining an oil with an acid, such as citrus or vinegar, and you can achieve specific flavor profiles by adding spices and fresh herbs. We recommend using a neutral-flavored oil, like avocado or olive oil. Part of making a vinaigrette is emulsifying the fat with the acid for a creamy dressing that won't separate. You do this by adding the oil to the acid slowly while mixing—easy to do in a blender.

¼ cup any vinegar or citrus juice
¾ cup Paleo-compliant oil

Add the vinegar or citrus juice to a blender. Blend on medium-low speed, and while the blender is running, slowly drizzle in the oil. Continue blending until the vinaigrette is smooth and uniformly combined, or emulsified. Transfer to an airtight jar with a lid and store for up to 2 weeks. If your mixture separates, or "breaks," don't worry—just stir or shake it to reincorporate. You can also make an intentionally "broken" vinaigrette by skipping the blender. Simply combine the ingredients in a jar with a lid and shake before using to combine.

Ingredient Swaps: Try incorporating fresh herbs for a bright and flavorful dressing. We recommend combining red wine vinegar with garlic, oregano, and Dijon mustard. Or, try a vinaigrette with lemon juice and sumac.

PER SERVING (2 TABLESPOONS): *Calories: 181; Total fat: 20g; Sodium: 1mg; Carbohydrates: 0g; Fiber: 0g; Protein: 0g; Iron: 0mg*

Spiced Maple Vinaigrette

» One-Pot, 5-Ingredient, 30 Minutes, Vegetarian

» Makes 1¼ cups

» Prep time: 5 minutes

This simple vinaigrette is a staple in our kitchens. It is quick and easy to throw together and works well on so many different salads. We like to pair it with sliced apples, shallots, fennel, and candied pecans. During colder months, enjoy it with Winter Squash Salad (page 74). This recipe uses smoked paprika (as opposed to regular sweet paprika) for an earthy, deep flavor.

½ cup apple cider vinegar

2 tablespoons smoked paprika

¼ cup maple syrup

½ cup extra-virgin olive oil

1. In a blender, combine the apple cider vinegar, paprika, and maple syrup. Blend on medium-low speed and, while the blender is running, slowly drizzle in the olive oil. Continue blending until the mixture emulsifies—it should look almost creamy.

2. Store the vinaigrette in an airtight container and keep refrigerated for up to 1 month.

Scale It Up: Double or triple this recipe to keep on hand for a quick lunch or dinner salad. The dressing keeps for 1 month but may separate over time—if it does, simply shake it before using to recombine.

PER SERVING (2 TABLESPOONS): *Calories: 122; Total fat: 11g; Sodium: 3mg; Carbohydrates: 6g; Fiber: 0g; Protein: 0g; Iron: 0mg*

Avocado-Cilantro Vinaigrette

» One-Pot, 5-Ingredient,
30-Minute, Low-Carb,
Diabetes-Friendly

» Makes 1½ cups

» Prep time: 10 minutes

With fresh cilantro and lime juice at center stage, this bright dressing with
heart-healthy avocado is perfect for a summer salad on a hot day. We originally developed this recipe to pair with Shrimp and Peach Salad (page 63), but it can be used in
many other dishes as well. Toss poached shrimp in this dressing and serve it with fresh
vegetables or use it as a sauce for roasted chicken.

1 large avocado, halved
and pitted
1 tablespoon plus
1 teaspoon lime juice
1 tablespoon water
1 tablespoon maple syrup
1 teaspoon sea salt
¼ teaspoon freshly ground
black pepper
2 teaspoons minced garlic
2 tablespoons olive oil
¼ cup chopped cilantro

Scoop the avocado flesh into a blender. Add the lime
juice, water, maple syrup, salt, pepper, and garlic. Blend
on medium speed for 2 minutes, or until smooth.
While the blender is running, slowly drizzle in the
olive oil. Stop the blender, add the cilantro, and pulse
5 times to incorporate. Adjust lime juice and water
to achieve desired consistency. Serve immediately or
refrigerate in an airtight container for up to 2 days.

Ingredient Swaps: For a slightly different flavor
profile, try replacing the cilantro with the same amount
of parsley.

PER SERVING (2 TABLESPOONS): *Calories: 112; Total fat: 10g; Sodium: 196mg; Carbohydrates: 7g;
Fiber: 3g; Protein: 1g; Iron: 0mg*

Paleo Mayo

» One-Pot, 5-Ingredient, 30 minutes, Low-Carb, Diabetes-Friendly, Vegetarian

» Makes 1½ cups

» Prep time: 10 minutes

Store-bought mayonnaise is typically made with soybean oil and is loaded with preservatives to prolong its shelf life. In other words, it is not Paleo-compliant. We developed this quick and super-versatile Paleo-friendly mayonnaise recipe you can make easily at home. Paleo Mayo will keep for up to 5 days in the refrigerator, but you'll use it often, so don't be afraid to make a full batch.

2 large egg yolks
1 tablespoon freshly squeezed lemon juice
2 teaspoons white wine vinegar
1 teaspoon mustard powder
½ teaspoon coconut sugar
1 teaspoon sea salt
1¼ cups olive oil

1. In a blender, combine the egg yolks, lemon juice, vinegar, mustard powder, coconut sugar, and salt. Blend on medium speed for 45 seconds, until light and airy and bright yellow in hue.

2. While the blender is running, slowly begin adding the olive oil, a few drops at a time to start. After about 1 minute of adding in drops, start drizzling the oil in a thin but steady stream, stopping occasionally to give the mixture a chance to emulsify. Continue pouring until all of the olive oil is incorporated—the mayonnaise should be thick. Keep refrigerated for up to 5 days in an airtight container.

Ingredient Swaps: If you don't have mustard powder, you can replace it with 1 teaspoon Dijon mustard.

PER SERVING (1 TABLESPOON): *Calories: 105; Total fat: 12g; Sodium: 49mg; Carbohydrates: 0g; Fiber: 0g; Protein: 0g; Iron: 0mg*

Nut-Free Pesto

» One-Pot, 30 Minutes, Low-Carb, Diabetes-Friendly, Vegetarian

» Makes 2 cups

» Prep time: 10 minutes

Pesto is a bright green sauce frequently seen in Italian cuisine and is typically made with basil, garlic, pine nuts, and Parmesan cheese. Although technically Paleo-friendly, pine nuts are a common allergy, so we use sunflower seeds instead to create a "pistou," or nut-free pesto. We also use nutritional yeast in place of Parmesan to maintain a rich, cheesy flavor. Use this pesto on Pesto Salmon (page 110) or as a spread on any sandwich.

2 cups fresh basil leaves

1 cup baby spinach leaves

½ cup olive oil

¼ cup toasted sunflower seeds

1 tablespoon nutritional yeast

1 tablespoon minced garlic

½ teaspoon sea salt

¼ teaspoon white pepper

In the bowl of a food processor or in a blender, combine the basil, spinach, olive oil, sunflower seeds, nutritional yeast, garlic, salt, and white pepper. Blend on medium speed for 2 minutes, stopping occasionally to scrape down the sides with a spatula. Continue blending until a loose paste forms. Transfer the pesto to an airtight container and keep refrigerated for up to 5 days.

Ingredient Swaps: The baby spinach in this recipe is optional—it offers vitamins and serves as a filler. If you don't have fresh spinach on hand, you can replace it with additional basil or fresh parsley.

PER SERVING (1/4 CUP): *Calories: 149; Total fat: 16g; Sodium: 77mg; Carbohydrates: 2g; Fiber: 1g; Protein: 1g; Iron: 1mg*

BBQ Sauce

» One-Pot, Vegetarian   » Makes 4 cups   » Prep time: 5 minutes
                                               Cook time: 35 minutes

Barbecue sauce is a crowd favorite—an entire genre of food exists around it. Unfortunately, most commercial barbecue sauces are packed with high-fructose corn syrup, so we created a Paleo version. Our BBQ Sauce is rich, healthy, and delicious, and you can adjust the spice level by adding or removing the chipotle peppers. Optional liquid smoke provides an easy way to achieve that smoky BBQ flavor without hours in the smoker.

1 tablespoon olive oil
1 (12-ounce) can
   tomato paste
½ cup honey
1 cup water
1 cup apple cider vinegar
1 tablespoon minced chipotle peppers in adobo
2 teaspoons kosher salt
2 teaspoons Dijon mustard
1 teaspoon garlic powder
½ teaspoon onion powder
½ teaspoon paprika
1 teaspoon liquid smoke
   (optional)

1. Heat the olive oil in a medium pot over medium-high heat. Add the tomato paste and cook, stirring frequently, for 2 minutes, until it is fragrant and starts to brown.

2. Add the honey, water, apple cider vinegar, chipotle peppers, salt, mustard, garlic powder, onion powder, paprika, and liquid smoke (if using). Bring the mixture to a boil, then reduce the heat to low. Simmer on low for 30 minutes, or until the sauce thickens. Using a whisk or hand mixer, vigorously blend the sauce until smooth.

3. Allow the sauce to cool to room temperature, then refrigerate it in an airtight container for up to 2 weeks.

Scale It Up: You can freeze this BBQ sauce in small portions. Thaw it in the refrigerator overnight before use. Double the recipe and divide the sauce into 1- or 2-person servings to freeze for easy use.

PER SERVING (2 TABLESPOONS): *Calories: 31; Total fat: 0g; Sodium: 83mg; Carbohydrates: 7g; Fiber: 1g; Protein: 1g; Iron: 0mg*

Tartar Sauce

» One-Pot, Low-Carb, Diabetes-Friendly, Vegetarian

» Makes 2 cups

» Prep time: 10 minutes, plus 1 hour to chill

Tartar sauce is mayonnaise-based and is usually served cold as an accompaniment to seafood. To brighten the flavor and add acidity in our Tartar Sauce, we use capers, lemon juice, and Refrigerator Dill Pickles. This sauce pairs well with grilled or fried fish, such as mahi-mahi or catfish. Try serving it with Seared Mahi-Mahi (page 103) in place of the Coconut-Caper Sauce, especially during hot summer months.

1 cup Paleo Mayo (page 156)

¼ cup Refrigerator Dill Pickles (page 49)

3 tablespoons capers, drained and minced

2 tablespoons chopped scallions

1 tablespoon minced shallot

1 tablespoon freshly squeezed lemon juice

1 tablespoon coarsely chopped parsley

1 teaspoon kosher salt

¼ teaspoon freshly ground black pepper

1. Prepare the mayo and dill pickles.

2. In a medium bowl, combine the mayo, pickles, capers, scallions, shallot, lemon juice, parsley, salt, and pepper. Mix by hand until all ingredients are incorporated. Cover and chill in the refrigerator for at least 1 hour before serving. Refrigerate in an airtight container for up to 5 days.

Make It Easier: Keeping batches of Paleo Mayo and Refrigerator Dill Pickles on hand will make this sauce quick and easy to throw together. If you are preparing them ahead, we recommend labeling them with the date they were made so you can keep track of how long they will stay fresh.

PER SERVING (2 TABLESPOONS): *Calories: 107; Total fat: 12g; Sodium: 149mg; Carbohydrates: 0g; Fiber: 0g; Protein: 0g; Iron: 0mg*

Guilt-Free Ranch Dressing

» One-Pot, 30 Minutes, Low-Carb, Diabetes-Friendly, Vegetarian

» Makes 2 cups

» Prep time: 10 minutes

Ranch dressing is one of the most popular salad dressings in the United States, but store-bought versions are loaded with trans fats and soybean oil, which are not Paleo-compliant. The base of this recipe uses Paleo Mayo (page 156) combined with nutritional yeast and spices for a healthy, rich, and creamy alternative to typical ranch. Serve this dressing on a salad or as a dipping sauce for Baked Buffalo Cauliflower (page 51).

1 cup Paleo Mayo (page 156)
1 cup full-fat coconut milk
1 teaspoon white wine vinegar
2 teaspoons nutritional yeast
1 tablespoon fresh minced dill
2 teaspoons fresh chopped chives
1 teaspoon onion powder
½ teaspoon garlic powder
¼ teaspoon freshly ground black pepper
1 teaspoon sea salt

1. Prepare the mayo.

2. In a large bowl, use a whisk or hand mixer to combine the mayo, coconut milk, white wine vinegar, and nutritional yeast until smooth.

3. Use a spoon to stir in the dill, chives, onion powder, garlic powder, pepper, and salt. Keep refrigerated in an airtight container for up to 1 week.

Make It Easier: Keeping a batch of Paleo Mayo on hand will make this sauce quick and easy to throw together for a salad or side. Paleo Mayo keeps for 5 days, so make it ahead to speed up prep time.

PER SERVING (2 TABLESPOONS): *Calories: 136; Total fat: 15g; Sodium: 124mg; Carbohydrates: 1g; Fiber: 0g; Protein: 0g; Iron: 1mg*

Thousand Island Dressing

» One-Pot, 5-Ingredient, 30 Minutes, Low-Carb, Diabetes-Friendly, Vegetarian

» Makes 1½ cups

» Prep time: 5 minutes
Cook time: 5 minutes, plus 1 hour to chill

Thousand Island dressing gets its name is supposed to have originated in the Thousand Islands region along the St. Lawrence River between the United States and Canada. This creamy, tangy dressing is a great way to use up extra Paleo Mayo (page 156), Zesty Ketchup (page 162), and Refrigerator Dill Pickles (page 49). Try it as an alternative to Russian dressing in Turkey Reuben Lettuce Wraps (page 94) or as a dip for Truffle Parsnip Fries (page 58).

1 cup Paleo Mayo (page 156)

2 tablespoons Zesty Ketchup (page 162)

2 tablespoons Refrigerator Dill Pickles (page 49), minced

2 tablespoons coconut aminos

1 tablespoon minced shallots

2 teaspoons coarsely chopped parsley

1 teaspoon sea salt

½ teaspoon garlic powder

¼ teaspoon freshly ground black pepper

¼ teaspoon paprika

1. If necessary, prepare the mayo, ketchup, and dill pickles.

2. In a medium bowl, combine the mayo, ketchup, dill pickles, coconut aminos, shallots, parsley, salt, garlic powder, pepper, and paprika. Whisk the ingredients until fully combined and refrigerate for 1 hour prior to serving. Store refrigerated for up to 6 days.

Ingredient Swaps: While we highly recommend keeping a batch of Zesty Ketchup on hand at all times, it can be substituted if you don't have it ready—simply replace the ketchup with 2 tablespoons tomato paste.

PER SERVING (1 TABLESPOON): *Calories: 171; Total fat: 19g; Sodium: 278mg; Carbohydrates: 0g; Fiber: 0g; Protein: 0g; Iron: 0mg*

Zesty Ketchup

» Vegetarian   » Makes 4 cups   » Prep time: 5 minutes
                                                 Cook time: 40 minutes

Ketchup is technically a tomato-based condiment, but store-bought versions often
have more high-fructose corn syrup and other sugars than they do tomato. This
large-batch homemade ketchup recipe uses healthy ingredients that children and
adults alike will enjoy. Don't skip the step of browning the tomato paste—this process
caramelizes its natural sugars, making the sauce smoother and sweeter.

2 tablespoons olive oil

1 cup small diced
   white onion

2 tablespoons
   tomato paste

1 (32-ounce) can whole
   peeled tomatoes

½ cup coconut sugar

½ cup apple cider vinegar

2 tablespoons
   minced garlic

1 teaspoon chili powder

½ teaspoon paprika

½ teaspoon allspice

¼ teaspoon cinnamon

1. Heat the olive oil in a large pot over medium-low heat.
   Add the onion and cook, stirring occasionally, until
   soft and translucent, about 5 minutes. Add the tomato
   paste and cook, stirring, for 2 to 3 minutes, until it
   starts to brown. Add the whole peeled tomatoes and
   stir, using a spatula to scrape up any browned bits from
   the bottom of the pot.

2. Add the coconut sugar, vinegar, garlic, chili powder,
   paprika, allspice, and cinnamon and stir to incorporate.
   Bring the mixture to a boil and then reduce the heat to
   low. Continue simmering for 25 to 30 minutes, stirring
   occasionally, until the mixture reduces and thickens.
   Remove from the heat.

3. Puree the ketchup in batches in a blender until
   smooth, or use an immersion blender to puree the
   sauce directly in the pot. The sauce will thicken as it
   cools, but if you want a thicker ketchup, return it to the
   pot and simmer for another 15 minutes over low heat.

4. Refrigerate the ketchup in an airtight container for up
   to 1 month or freeze for up to 3 months.

Scale It Up: Double or even triple this recipe to keep
your refrigerator stocked with this staple ingredient.

PER SERVING (1 TABLESPOON): *Calories: 15; Total fat: 0g; Sodium: 18mg; Carbohydrates: 3g;
Fiber: 0g; Protein: 0g; Iron: 0mg*

Honey Mustard Sauce

» One-Pot, 5-Ingredient, Vegetarian   » Makes ¾ cup   » Prep time: 5 minutes

Honey mustard is a staple condiment at countless restaurants. Unfortunately, many honey mustard sauces are loaded with added sugars and preservatives and therefore are not Paleo-compliant. This is our quick and easy recipe for Paleo-friendly Honey Mustard. Try serving this sauce with grilled chicken, pork tenderloin, or as a dressing for your next salad.

½ cup raw honey
¼ cup Dijon mustard
2 tablespoons
  yellow mustard
¼ teaspoon sea salt
⅛ teaspoon white pepper

In a small mixing bowl, combine the honey, Dijon mustard, yellow mustard, salt, and pepper. Whisk thoroughly until all ingredients are combined. Enjoy immediately or refrigerate in an airtight container for up to 1 month.

Scale It Up: Since this sauce keeps for up to 1 month, we recommend doubling or tripling it so you always have it at the ready.

PER SERVING (2 TABLESPOONS): *Calories: 95; Total fat: 1g; Sodium: 198mg; Carbohydrates: 24g; Fiber: 1g; Protein: 1g; Iron: 0mg*

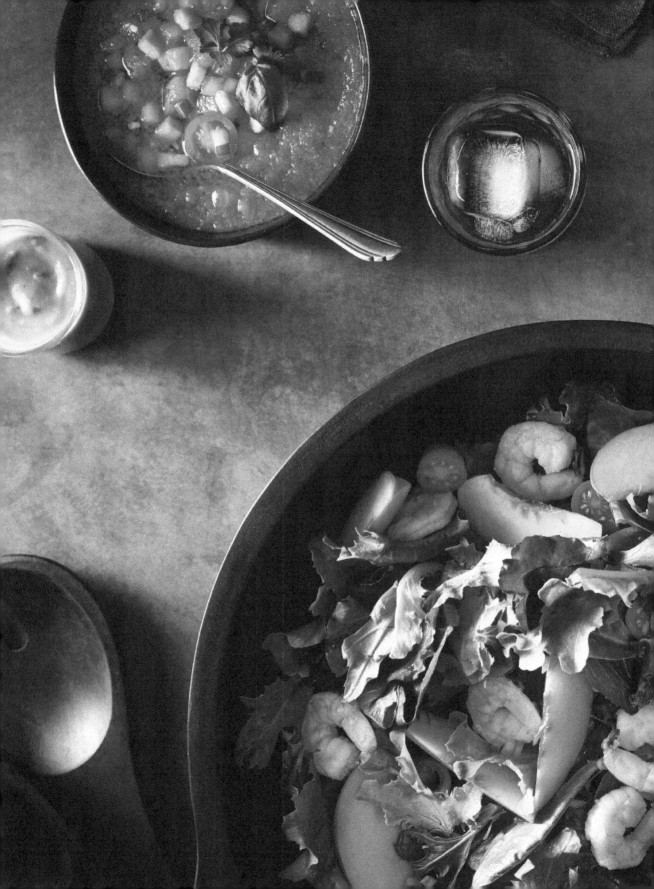

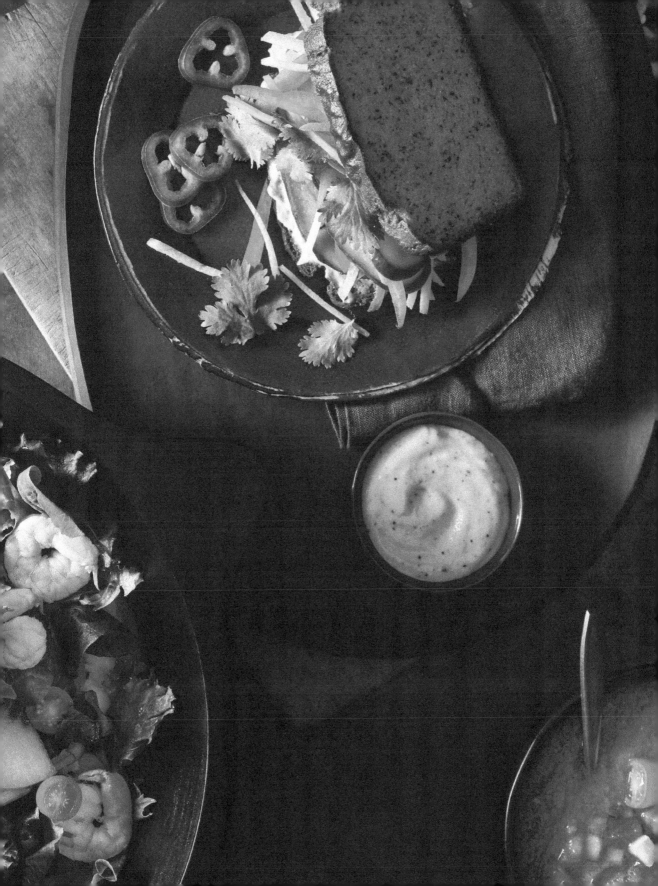

Measurement Conversions

Volume Equivalents	U.S. Standard	U.S. Standard (OUNCES)	Metric (APPROXIMATE)
Liquid	2 tablespoons	1 fl. oz.	30 mL
	¼ cup	2 fl. oz.	60 mL
	½ cup	4 fl. oz.	120 mL
	1 cup	8 fl. oz.	240 mL
	1½ cups	12 fl. oz.	355 mL
	2 cups or 1 pint	16 fl. oz.	475 mL
	4 cups or 1 quart	32 fl. oz.	1 L
	1 gallon	128 fl. oz.	4 L
Dry	⅛ teaspoon	–	0.5 mL
	¼ teaspoon	–	1 mL
	½ teaspoon	–	2 mL
	¾ teaspoon	–	4 mL
	1 teaspoon	–	5 mL
	1 tablespoon	–	15 mL
	¼ cup	–	59 mL
	⅓ cup	–	79 mL
	½ cup	–	118 mL
	⅔ cup	–	156 mL
	¾ cup	–	177 mL
	1 cup	–	235 mL
	2 cups or 1 pint	–	475 mL
	3 cups	–	700 mL
	4 cups or 1 quart	–	1 L
	½ gallon	–	2 L
	1 gallon	–	4 L

Oven Temperatures

Fahrenheit	Celsius (APPROXIMATE)
250°F	120°C
300°F	150°C
325°F	165°C
350°F	180°C
375°F	190°C
400°F	200°C
425°F	220°C
450°F	230°C

Weight Equivalents

U.S. Standard	Metric (APPROXIMATE)
½ ounce	15 g
1 ounce	30 g
2 ounces	60 g
4 ounces	115 g
8 ounces	225 g
12 ounces	340 g
16 ounces or 1 pound	455 g

Resources

The following books and websites are great sources for learning about and cooking to adhere to the Paleo diet:

» *The Paleo Mom* (blog) by Dr. Sarah Ballantyne (ThePaleoMom.com)

» *Grain Brain: The Surprising Truth About Wheat, Carbs, and Sugar* by David Perlmutter

» *The Paleo Approach: Reverse Autoimmune Disease and Heal Your Body* by Dr. Sarah Ballantyne

» *Primal Body, Primal Mind: Beyond the Paleo Diet for Total Health and a Longer Life* by Nora Gedgaudas

» *Against All Grain* (blog) by Danielle Walker AgainstAllGrain.com

» *The Food Lover's Companion* by Sharon Tyler Herbst

» *The Food Lab: Better Home Cooking Through Science* by J. Kenji López-Alt

» *100 Techniques: Master a Lifetime of Cooking Skills, from Basic to Bucket List* by America's Test Kitchen

» *Eat Dirt: Why Leaky Gut May Be the Root Cause of Your Health Problems and 5 Surprising Steps to Cure It* by Josh Axe

» *The Flavor Bible* by Andrew Dornenburg and Karen A. Page

Index

Acknowledgments

We would like to thank our friends, family, coworkers, and loyal customers for their support while writing this book. We could not have achieved any of this without you all!

About the Authors

 Ashley Ramirez, PhD, founder of Mason Dixon Bakery & Bistro, learned she had celiac disease while in college. She went on to receive her doctorate in chemistry from Duke University in 2012. After receiving her degree, she relocated to Alabama, where a series of serendipitous events led to the creation of Mason Dixon. She dreamed of using her background in science to develop gluten-free recipes to win over even the toughest critics. Her passion for healthy living and providing for her community continues to drive her business every day.

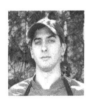 **Matthew Streeter** has been a part of Alabama's culinary scene since 2004. Growing up in a military family, frequent traveling helped introduce him to cuisines from around the world. His passion and curiosity for foods from around the world shines through in the dishes he creates. In 2014, Matthew helped open the bistro side of Mason Dixon, a dedicated gluten-free and Paleo-friendly restaurant. Over the years, he has shown that healthy and allergen-free food can be delicious, complex, and satisfying.

CPSIA information can be obtained
at www.ICGtesting.com
Printed in the USA
JSHW010837181120
9469JS00007B/11

9 781647 397357